Clinical Ophthalmology
A self-assessment companion

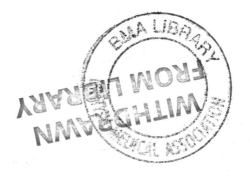

For Elsevier:

Commissioning Editor: Robert Edwards
Development Editor: Rebecca Gleave
Project Manager: Frances Affleck
Design Direction: Stewart Larking
Page Design: Lee-May Lim

Clinical Ophthalmology
A self-assessment companion

By **Jack J. Kanski MD MS FRCS FRCOphth**
Honorary Consultant Ophthalmic Surgeon,
Prince Charles Eye Unit,
King Edward VII Hospital, Windsor, UK.

Agnes Kubicka-Trząska MD
Senior Lecturer,
Department of Ophthalmology,
Jagiellonian University, Kraków, Poland

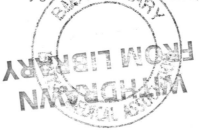

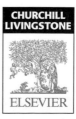

CHURCHILL LIVINGSTONE

ELSEVIER

Edinburgh London New York Oxford Philadelphia St Louis Sydney Toronto 2007

First published 2007

ISBN 0750675381
ISBN 13 9780750675383

British Library Cataloguing in Publication Data
A catalogue record for this book is available from the British Library

Library of Congress Cataloging in Publication Data
A catalog record for this book is available from the Library of Congress

Note
Knowledge and best practice in this field are constantly changing. As new research and experience broaden our knowledge, changes in practice, treatment and drug therapy may become necessary or appropriate. Readers are advised to check the most current information provided (i) on procedures featured or (ii) by the manufacturer of each product to be administered, to verify the recommended dose or formula, the method and duration of administration, and contraindications. It is the responsibility of the practitioner, relying on their own experience and knowledge of the patient, to make diagnoses, to determine dosages and the best treatment for each individual patient, and to take all appropriate safety precautions. To the fullest extent of the law, neither the publisher nor the editors assume any liability for any injury and/or damage.

The Publisher

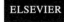

your source for books,
journals and multimedia
in the health sciences

www.elsevierhealth.com

Working together to grow
libraries in developing countries

www.elsevier.com | www.bookaid.org | www.sabre.org

ELSEVIER   BOOK AID   Sabre Foundation
            International

The
publisher's
policy is to use
**paper manufactured
from sustainable forests**

Printed in China

Contents

Preface

The main object of this book is to help those preparing
for postgraduate examinations in ophthalmology. *Self-
assessment Companion* is designed to be used in conjunction
with *Clinical Ophthalmology* 6th edition which contains
24 corresponding chapters.

Most questions have six stems that require either a direct
answer or a true or false answer, for those in multiple
choice format. The majority of the images are different from
those in *Clinical Ophthalmology* and are intended to act as
clues to a question or to reinforce the reader's knowledge
of a particular topic. Systematic use of this book should
indicate to the reader areas requiring further study. It is
suggested that a chapter in *Clinical Ophthalmology* is read
first and then the reader uses this book for self-assessment
on a particular section. The last chapter in this book is a
referral guide for optometrists.

J.J.K. and A.K-T.

Acknowledgements

We are very grateful to the colleagues and ophthalmic photographers listed below for generously supplying us with additional images:

S. Barabino, C. Barry, P. Curi, R. Curtis, B. Damato, the Eye Academy, C. de A. Garcia, A. Garner, P. Gili, J. Harry, L. Horton, S. Kumar Puri, M. Leyland, A. Leys, W. Lisch, L. MacKeen, L. Merin, S. Milenkovic, S. Milewski, M. Mir, S. Mitchell, A. Moore, Moorfields Eye Hospital, K. Nischal, B. Noble, M. Parulekar, C. Pavésio, A. Pearson, E. Pringle, U. Raina, N. Rogers, P. Saine, M. Sanders, J. Sloper, S. Tuft, P. Watts and J. Yangüela.

We are also greatly indebted to Aasheet Desai for meticulously reviewing the manuscript.

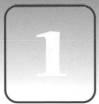

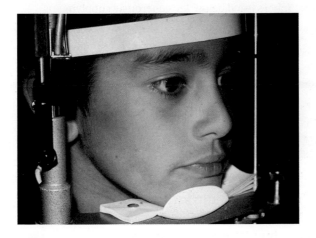

1 **Q. What are the main methods of slit-lamp biomicroscopy of the cornea?**

A.

a. Direct illumination with diffuse light to detect gross abnormalities.

b. Scleral scatter involves decentring the slit beam laterally so that the light is incident on the limbus with the microscope focused centrally.

c. Retroillumination uses reflected light from the iris or fundus.

d. Specular reflection shows abnormalities of the endothelium such as reduced cell density and guttata.

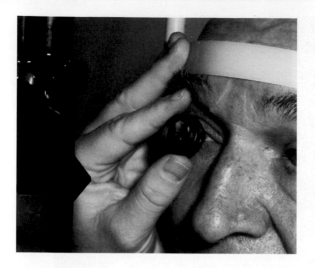

2   Q. Indirect slit-lamp biomicroscopy – true or false?

a. The image is vertically inverted and laterally reversed.
b. The slit beam is adjusted to a width about $^1/_2$ of its full round diameter.
c. The illumination is set at an angle coaxial with the slit-lamp viewing system.
d. The magnification and light intensity are adjusted to the highest settings.
e. The light beam should be centred to pass directly through the pupil.
f. The fundus is examined by moving the lens into the appropriate positions.

A.
a. True. **b.** False – $^1/_4$ **c.** True. **d.** False – lowest. **e.** True. **f.** False – lens is kept still and the joystick and vertical adjustments are moved.

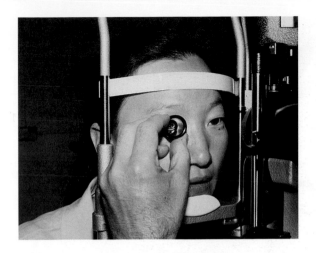

3 Q. Goldmann three-mirror examination – true or false?

a. The curvature of the cornea is steeper than that of the goniolens.

b. Viscous coupling substance has the same refractive index as the cornea.

c. The large oblong mirror enables visualization between the equator and ora serrata.

d. The dome-shaped mirror may be used to visualize the extreme fundus periphery.

e. When viewing the vertical meridian the image is upside down and laterally reversed.

f. The illumination column should always be tilted except when viewing the 12 o'clock position in the fundus (i.e. with the mirror at 6 o'clock).

A.

a. False – goniolens curvature is steeper than that of the cornea. **b.** True. **c.** False – between 30° and the equator. **d.** True. **e.** False – upside down, but not laterally reversed. **f.** True.

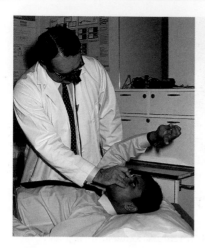

4 Q. Indirect ophthalmoscopy – true or false?

a. An inverted and laterally reversed image of the fundus is provided.

b. As the power of the condensing lens decreases, the working distance and the magnification increase, but the field of view is reduced and vice versa.

c. 20D lens magnifies x 3.

d. 30D lens has a longer working distance than a 15D lens.

e. When performing scleral indentation the indenter should be kept perpendicular with the globe.

f. Lattice degeneration is drawn as blue hatchings outlined in red.

A.

a. True. **b.** True. **c.** True. **d.** False – shorter. **e.** False – tangential to the globe. **f.** False – outlined in blue not red.

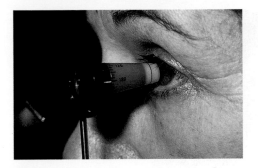

5   Q. Tonometry – true or false?

a. The Imbert–Fick principle states that for an ideal, dry, thin-walled sphere, the pressure inside the sphere (P) equals the force necessary to flatten its surface (F) divided by the area of flattening (A) (i.e. P=F/A).

b. In Goldmann tonometry (see above) corneal rigidity and capillary attraction cancel each other when the flattened area has a diameter of 3.60 mm.

c. Corneal oedema may result in an artificially high reading.

d. The normal central corneal thickness is assumed to be 550 μm.

e. Patients with ocular hypertension tend to have thinner corneas.

f. Following laser refractive surgery intraocular pressure may be underestimated.

A.

a. True. **b.** False – 3.06 mm. **c.** False – low. **d.** True. **e.** False – thicker. **f.** True.

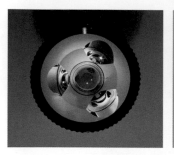 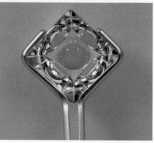

6   Q. Goniolenses – true or false?

a. The Goldmann (see above left) is a direct goniolens with a contact surface diameter of approximately 12 mm.

b. The Goldmann does not require a coupling fluid.

c. The Zeiss (see above right) is an indirect goniolens.

d. The Zeiss goniolens has a diameter of 9 mm and a curvature flatter than that of the cornea.

e. The Zeiss goniolens requires a coupling fluid.

f. The Zeiss goniolens is suitable for laser trabeculoplasty.

A.

a. False – indirect. **b.** False. **c.** True. **d.** True. **e.** False. **f.** False.

7 Q. Gonioscopy – true or false?

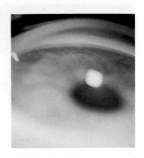

a. In Goldmann gonioscopy (see right) the image is laterally reversed with the mirror in the horizontal meridian and vertically inverted when in the vertical meridian.

b. The Goldmann goniolens is suitable for indentation gonioscopy.

c. During Zeiss gonioscopy the patient must look straight ahead.

d. The angle in Shaffer grade 3 is incapable of closure.

e. In a Shaffer grade 4 the apex of the corneal wedge cannot be visualized.

f. Trabecular pigmentation in normal eyes is most marked in the anterior trabeculum and superiorly.

g. Schwalbe line represents peripheral termination of Descemet membrane and anterior limit of the trabeculum.

h. The trabeculum has an average width of 800 μm.

i. Blood in Schlemm canal is always pathological.

j. Iris processes are more prominent in children.

k. The ciliary body band tends to be narrower in myopic eyes.

A.

a. True. **b.** False. **c.** True. **d.** True. **e.** False. **f.** False – posterior trabeculum and inferiorly. **g.** True. **h.** False – 600 μm. **i.** False. **j.** True. **k.** False – broader.

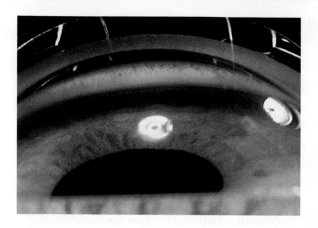

8   Q. Blood in Schlemm canal may occur in the following – true or false?

a. Carotid-cavernous fistula.

b. Sturge–Weber syndrome.

c. Ghost-cell glaucoma.

d. Obstruction of the superior vena cava.

e. Ocular hypotony.

f. Polycythaemia.

A.

a. True. **b.** True. **c.** False. **d.** True. **e.** True. **f.** False.

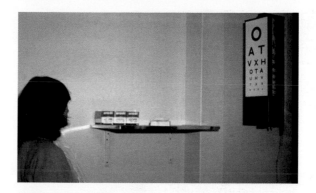

9 Q. Visual acuity charts – answer the following.

a. In the Snellen chart (see above) how much (in minutes of arc) does the $^6/_6$ letter subtend at 6 m?

b. In the Snellen chart how much (in minutes of arc) does the $^6/_{60}$ letter subtend at 6 m?

c. What is $^6/_{12}$ expressed as a decimal?

d. In macular disease is visual acuity better or worse when looking through a pin hole?

e. What does MAR stand for?

f. How many letters are there in each row of the Bailey–Lovie chart?

A.

a. 5 minutes of arc. **b.** 50 minutes of arc. **c.** 0.5. **d.** Worse. **e.** Minimum angle of resolution. **f.** 5 letters.

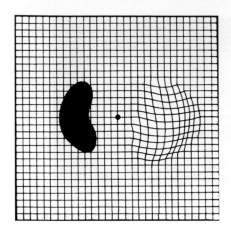

10   Q. Amsler grid – answer the following.

a. What is the purpose of the test?

b. How much of the visual field does the grid assess?

c. How many squares does chart number 1 contain?

d. What is the angle subtended by each small square in chart number 1?

e. How does chart number 3 differ from chart number 1?

f. Which chart is the most sensitive?

A.

a. To detect a central visual field defect or metamorphopsia (see above).

b. 20%. **c.** 400 squares. **d.** One degree of visual angle. **e.** The squares are red and not white. **f.** Chart number 7 because it contains a fine central grid.

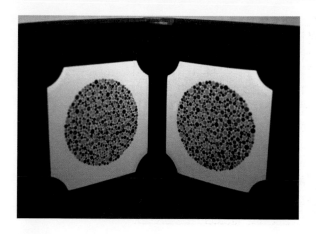

11 Q. Colour vision testing – answer the following.

a. What is the most common congenital colour vision defect?

b. What is a protanomalous trichromat?

c. How many plates does the Ishihara test contain (see above)?

d. What is the configuration of each Ishihara plate?

e. How many colours does each plate of the City University test contain?

f. How is the City University test performed?

A.

a. Anomalous trichromatism. **b.** A red–green deficient individual who has an abnormality of red-sensitive cones. **c.** 17 – one of which is a test plate to detect malingering. **d.** A matrix of pseudo-isochromatic dots arranged to show a central shape or number which the subject is asked to identify. **e.** 5 – one central and four peripheral. **f.** The subject is asked to select one of the peripheral colours which most closely match the central colour.

12 Q. Dark adaptometry – answer the following.

a. Define the phenomenon of dark adaptation.

b. What is the main indication for dark adaptometry?

c. What percentage of rhodopsin is bleached when the patient is exposed to bright light in the Goldmann–Weekes test?

d. What does the cone branch of the sensitivity curve represent?

e. In normal subjects when does the 'rod-cone' break occur?

f. What does the rod branch of the curve represent?

A.

a. The phenomenon by which the visual system (pupil, retina and occipital cortex) adapts to decreased illumination. **b.** Investigation of patients complaining of night-blindness (nyctalopia). **c.** 25% or more. **d.** The initial 5–10 minutes of darkness during which cone sensitivity rapidly improves. **e.** After 7–10 minutes when cones achieve their maximum sensitivity and the rods become perceptibly more sensitive than cones. **f.** The continuation of improvement of rod sensitivity.

13   Q. Electroretinography – true or false?

a. The reference electrode is embedded in a contact lens and the active electrode on the forehead.

b. The a-wave is the initial fast-negative deflection.

c. The amplitude of the b-wave is measured from the peak of the a-wave to the trough of the b-wave.

d. The b2 subcomponent of the b-wave represents mainly cone activity.

e. Combined rod and cone responses are elicited with a very bright white flash resulting in a prominent a-wave and a b-wave.

f. Cone flicker is used to isolate cones by using a flickering light stimulus at a frequency of 30 Hz to which rods cannot respond.

A.

a. False – reverse applies. **b.** True. **c.** False – trough of the a-wave to the peak of the b-wave. **d.** True. **e.** True. **f.** True.

14 Q. Electro-oculography – true or false?

a. It measures the standing potential between the electrically negative cornea and the electrically positive back of the eye.

b. Electrodes are attached to the skin near the medial and lateral canthi.

c. It may be used to assess macular function.

d. It is normal in optic atrophy.

e. It may be abnormal in advanced chloroquine retinotoxicity.

f. The normal ratio is over 1.5 (150%).

A.

a. False – reverse applies. **b.** True. **c.** False. **d.** True. **e.** True. **f.** False – over 1.85 (185%).

15 Q. Visual-evoked potential – true or false?

a. It is a recording of electrical activity of the visual cortex created by stimulation of the retina.

b. It is not an appropriate investigation in infants.

c. Pattern visual-evoked potential is elicited by a flash of light.

d. In optic neuropathy it shows prolonged latency and decreased amplitude.

e. Latency varies in normal subjects 2–5% within and between recording sessions.

f. Absolute amplitude is more reliable than absolute latency.

A.

a. True. **b.** False. **c.** False – checker-board pattern. **d.** True. **e.** True.
f. False – reverse applies.

16   Q. Define the following perimetric terms.

a. Isopter.
b. Relative scotoma.
c. Luminance.
d. Decibel (dB).
e. Differential light sensitivity.
f. Visible threshold.

A.

a. A contour line on a map that encloses an area within which a target of a given size is visible. **b.** Area of partial visual loss within which brighter or larger targets can be seen and smaller or dimmer ones cannot.
c. Intensity or 'brightness' of a light stimulus, measured in apostilb (asb).
d. Non-specific unit of luminance based on a logarithmic scale (one-tenth of a log unit). **e.** Degree by which the luminance of a target requires to exceed background luminance in order to be perceived by the eye.
f. Luminance of a given stimulus (measured in asb or dB) at which it is perceived 50% of the time when presented statically.

17 Q. Perimetry – true or false?

a. Perimetry involves evaluation of the visual field.

b. Kinetic perimetry is a three-dimensional assessment of the boundary of the hill of vision.

c. Kinetic perimetry involves the presentation of a moving stimulus of known luminance or intensity from a non-seeing area to a seeing area until it is perceived.

d. Static perimetry involves the presentation of non-moving stimuli of varying luminance in the same position to obtain a vertical boundary of the visual field.

e. Static perimetry can be performed by confrontation.

f. Threshold perimetry involves presentation of visual stimuli at luminance levels above expected normal threshold values in various locations of the visual field.

A.

a. True. **b.** False – two-dimensional. **c.** True. **d.** True. **e.** False. **f.** False – suprathreshold perimetry.

18 Q. Define the following terms in Humphrey perimetry.

a. Total deviation.

b. Pattern deviation.

c. Reliability indices.

d. Global indices.

e. Pattern standard deviation.

f. Corrected pattern standard deviation.

A.

a. Deviation of the patient's result from that of age-matched controls.
b. This is similar to total deviation, except that it is adjusted for any generalized depression in the overall field that might be caused by other factors, such as lens opacities or miosis. **c.** Extent to which the patient's results are reliable and should be analyzed first. If grossly unreliable, further evaluation of a visual field printout is pointless. **d.** A summary of the results in a single number, principally used to monitor progression of glaucomatous damage rather than for initial diagnosis. **e.** Measure of focal loss or variability within the field, taking into account any generalized depression in the hill of vision. **f.** Measure of variability within the field after correcting for short-term fluctuation (intra-test variability).

19 Q. Humphrey perimetry – true or false?

a. Background luminance of 31.5 asb and target luminance can be varied between 0.08 asb and 10 000 asb brighter than background, which equates to a decibel range of 51–0.

b. It is suitable only for threshold perimetry.

c. The 24° strategy tests 54 points and the 30° strategy tests 76 points.

d. A fixation loss is detected when a stimulus is accompanied by a sound.

e. The greyscale printout in individuals with high false-positive responses has a clover leaf shape.

f. The standard SITA strategy is more sensitive than full-threshold perimetry in detecting early visual field loss.

A.

a. True. **b.** False – suprathreshold perimetry. **c.** True. **d.** False. **e.** False – high false-negative. **f.** True.

20 Q. Match the visual field defect (a–f) with the appropriate condition (i–vi).

a. Unilateral inferior altitudinal.

b. Bilateral ring scotomas.

c. Unilateral centrocaecal scotoma.

d. Unilateral central scotoma.

e. Bilateral paracentral scotomas.

f. Severe bilateral constriction ('tunnel' vision).

i. Anterior ischaemic optic neuropathy.

ii. Retrobulbar neuritis.

iii. Glaucoma.

iv. Hysteria.

v. Leber hereditary optic neuropathy.

vi. Retinitis pigmentosa.

A.

a. & **i**; **b.** & **vi**; **c.** & **v**; **d.** & **ii**; **e.** & **iii**; **f.** & **iv**.

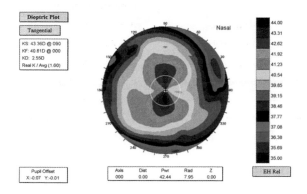

1 Q. Corneal imaging – true or false?

a. Normal cell density is about 4000 cells/mm^2.

b. Corneal oedema is likely to occur following cataract surgery when the endothelial cell count is 500 cells/mm^2.

c. Specular microscopy is of no value in evaluating donor corneal tissue.

d. In corneal topography steep curvatures are coloured orange and red.

e. In corneal topography flat curvatures are coloured violet and blue.

f. In corneal topography an absolute scale should not be used for comparison over time.

A.

a. False – 3000 cells/mm^2. **b.** True. **c.** False. **d.** True (see above). **e.** True.
f. False.

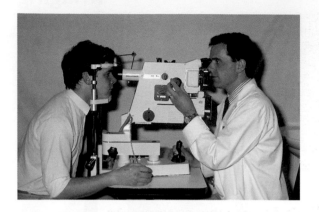

2   Q. Fluorescein angiography – define the following.

a. Fluorescein.

b. Fluorescence.

c. Fluorescein angiography.

d. Fluorescein binding.

e. Outer blood–retinal barrier.

f. Inner blood–retinal barrier.

A.

a. Orange water-soluble dye that remains largely intravascular and circulates in the blood stream. **b.** Property of certain molecules to emit light of a longer wavelength when stimulated by light of a shorter wavelength. **c.** Photographic surveillance of the passage of fluorescein through the retinal and choroidal circulations following intravenous injection. **d.** On intravenous injection, 70–85% of fluorescein molecules bind to serum proteins (bound fluorescein); the remainder remain unbound (free fluorescein). **e.** Tight junctional intercellular complexes in the RPE termed zonula occludens. **f.** Tight junctions between retinal capillary endothelial cells.

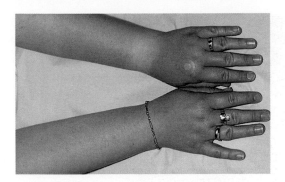

3   Q. Fluorescein angiography – true or false?

a. The excitation peak for fluorescein is about 530 nm.
b. Blue light enters the eye and yellow-green light enters the camera.
c. The usual amount of fluorescein used is 3 ml of a 25% solution.
d. Images are taken at one second intervals for 5–25 seconds after injection.
e. A late image is always taken after 20 minutes.
f. Urticaria (see above) is a common side-effect.

A.

a. False – 490 nm. **b.** True. **c.** False – 5 ml of a 10% solution. **d.** True.
e. False – only if leakage is anticipated. **f.** False – rare.

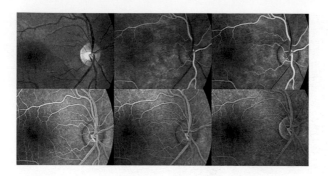

4 **Q. Describe the main phases of a fluorescein angiogram.**

A.

a. The choroidal (pre-arterial) phase occurs 8–12 seconds after the dye injection and is characterized by patchy filling of the choroid due to leakage of free fluorescein through the fenestrated choriocapillaris. b. The arterial phase which shows arterial filling and the continuation of choroidal filling. c. The arteriovenous (capillary) phase shows complete filling of the arteries and capillaries with early laminar flow in the veins. d. The venous phase which can be subdivided into: the *early* phase exhibits complete arterial and capillary filling, and more marked laminar venous flow; the *mid* phase displays almost complete venous filling; the *late* phase shows complete venous filling with reducing concentration of dye in the arteries. e. The late (elimination) phase demonstrates the effects of continuous recirculation, dilution and elimination of the dye.

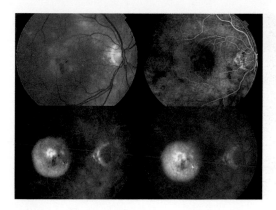

5 Q. Appearance on fluorescein angiography – true or false?

a. The dark appearance of the fovea is partly caused by blockage of background choroidal fluorescence due to increased density of xanthophyll at the fovea.

b. A transmission defect is caused by focal atrophy of the choriocapillaris.

c. A transmission defect is characterized by early hyperfluorescence which increases in intensity and then fades without changing in size or shape.

d. Pooling in the subretinal space is characterized by early hyperfluorescence which increases in intensity but not in size.

e. Pooling in the sub-RPE space is characterized by early hyperfluorescence which increases in intensity but not in size.

f. A choroidal naevus may block background choroidal fluorescence.

A.

a. True. **b.** False – atrophy of the RPE. **c.** True. **d.** False – hyperfluorescence increases in size. **e.** True (see above). **f.** True.

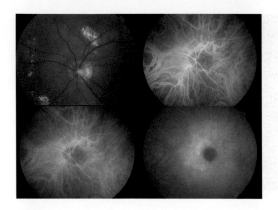

6   Q. Indocyanine green angiography – true or false?

a. It is not useful in delineating the choroidal circulation.

b. About 98% of molecules bind to albumin.

c. The emission is at 835 nm.

d. A retinal pigment epithelial window defect shows hypofluorescence.

e. A retinal pigment epithelial detachment shows hypofluorescence.

f. It is very useful in demonstrating polypoidal choroidal vasculopathy.

A.

a. False. b. True. c. True. d. False e. True. f. True.

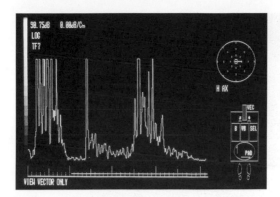

7 Q. Define the following ultrasonographic terms.

a. Ultrasound.

b. Ultrasonography.

c. Transducer.

d. A-scan ultrasonography.

e. High-frequency ultrasonography.

f. Gain.

A.

a. Sound that is beyond the range of human hearing. **b.** Ultrasonography uses high frequency sound waves to produce echoes as they strike interfaces between acoustically distinct structures. **c.** Piezoelectric crystal which when stimulated with an electric current vibrates at such a frequency as to emit ultrasonic waves. **d.** A-scan ultrasonography is performed with a single ultrasound source. It produces a one-dimensional time–amplitude evaluation in the form of vertical spikes along a baseline (see above). **e.** High-frequency B-scan ultrasonography utilizes 30–50 MHz and allows high-definition imaging of the anterior segment but only to a depth of 5 mm. **f.** Adjustment of the amplification of the echo signal, similar to volume control of a radio.

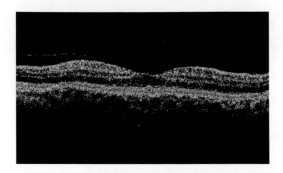

8   Q. Optical coherence tomography (OCT) – true or false?

a. It is analogous to B-scan ultrasonography but uses light instead of sound waves.

b. Measurements are performed by directing a beam of light and measuring the echo time delay and magnitude of reflected or backscattering light using low-coherence interferometry.

c. It is useful in detecting vitreomacular traction.

d. It is not useful in measuring retinal thickness.

e. It cannot differentiate retinoschisis from retinal detachment.

f. Ultrahigh resolution OCT can identify the internal limiting membrane.

A.

a. True. b. True. c. True. d. False. e. False f. True.

9 Q. Describe the display of the Heidelberg Retinal Tomograph (HRT).

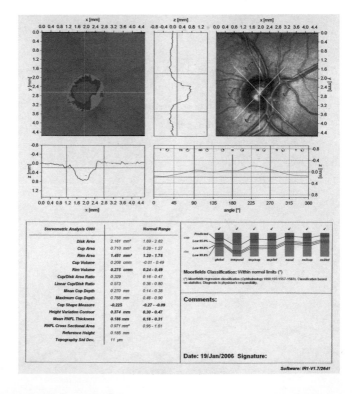

A.

a. In the topographic image (top left) the cup is represented in red, the neuroretinal rim in green and the slope in blue. **b.** The reflectivity image (top right) is divided into six sectors. A green tick within a sector indicates within normal limits, a yellow exclamation mark borderline and a red cross abnormal. **c.** The two cross-section images (top centre and middle left) show the amount of cupping in the vertical and horizontal planes. **d.** The graph (centre right) displays the height variation of the retinal surface along the contour line (green). **e.** The Moorfields regression analysis is depicted as a seven-colour bar graph, one bar for each segment and one global bar (bottom right). **f.** Detailed stereometric data are presented in a table (bottom left). Readings outside normal are indicated with an asterisk.

10 Q. Describe the display of the GDxVCC.

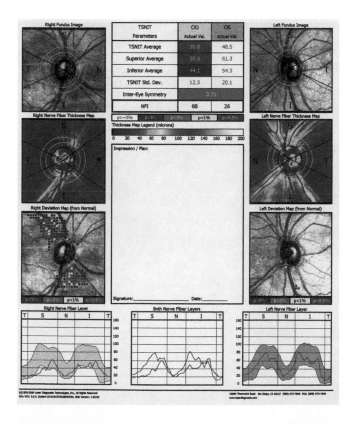

A.

The display provides colour images of the optic nerve head and retinal nerve fibre (RNF) maps in the four quadrants. **a.** The fundus image of the left and right eyes at the top is useful in identifying image quality. **b.** The thickness maps are presented in a colour-coded spectrum from blue to red. **c.** The deviation maps show the location and magnitude of RNF defects as tiny colour codes squares (pixels). **d.** The TSNIT (temporal-superior-nasal-inferior-temporal) graph is displayed at the bottom. It shows the actual values for that eye along with a shaded area that represents the 95% normal range for that age. **e.** Parameters for each eye are displayed in a table (top centre). **f.** The nerve fibre indicator (NFI) at the bottom of the table indicates a global value based on the entire thickness map and is the optimal parameter for discriminating normal from glaucoma.

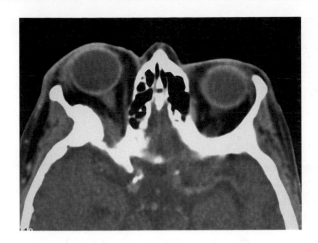

11 Q. Computed tomography – true or false?

a. It is not well tolerated by claustrophobic patients.

b. Dense structures appear dark and minimally dense structures appear white.

c. Contrast is indicated in the assessment of acute haemorrhage.

d. It exposes the patient to ionizing radiation.

e. It may be used to detect optic disc drusen.

f. It is safe to use in patients with ferrous foreign bodies.

A.

a. False. **b.** False – dense structures are white (see above). **c.** False – contraindicated. **d.** True. **e.** True. **f.** True.

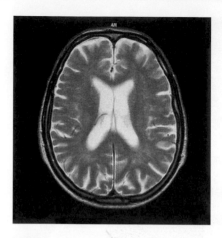

12   Q. Magnetic resonance imaging – true or false?

a. Bone appears black.

b. T2-weighted images are best for demonstrating normal anatomy.

c. In T1-weighted images vitreous is hypointense and fat is hyperintense.

d. Gadolinium is used only in T1-weighted imaging.

e. It is not suitable for detecting enlarged extraocular muscles.

f. STIR images have a have very low signal from fat but still have high signal from water.

A.

a. True (see above). **b.** False. **c.** True. **d.** True. **e.** False. **f.** True.

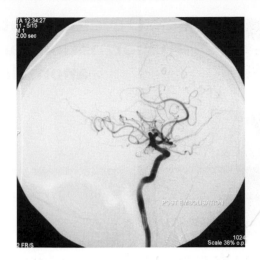

13 Q. Neuro-angiography – true or false?

a. Magnetic resonance angiography (MRA) requires contrast.

b. MRA may miss very small aneurysms.

c. Magnetic resonance venography is used to diagnose venous sinus thrombosis.

d. Computed tomography angiography (CTA) carries a 1% risk of stroke.

e. CTA is the method of choice for investigation of intracranial aneurysms.

f. Conventional intra-arterial angiography (see above) requires a general anaesthetic.

A.

a. False. b. True. c. True. d. False. e. True. f. False.

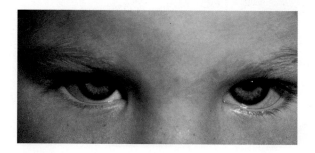

1 Q. Epicanthic folds – true or false?

a. Epicanthic folds may give rise to pseudo-exotropia.

b. Epicanthus tarsalis in the most common type in Orientals.

c. Epicanthus inversus is associated with the blepharophimosis syndrome.

d. Epicanthus tarsalis is the most common type in Caucasians.

e. Small folds may require Y–V plasty.

f. Large folds may require skin grafts.

A.

a. False – pseudo-esotropia (see above). **b.** True. **c.** True. **d.** False – Orientals. **e.** True. **f.** False – Mustarde Z-plasty.

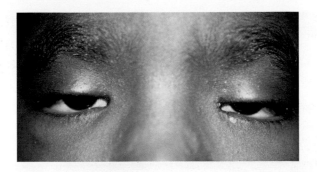

2   **Q. Blepharophimosis syndrome is characterized by the following except – true or false?**

a. Moderate-to-severe symmetrical ptosis.

b. Good levator function.

c. Short horizontal palpebral aperture.

d. Telecanthus.

e. Lateral ectropion of lower lids.

f. Amblyopia in 50% of cases.

A.

a. True. **b.** False – levator function is poor. **c.** True. **d.** True. **e.** True.

f. True.

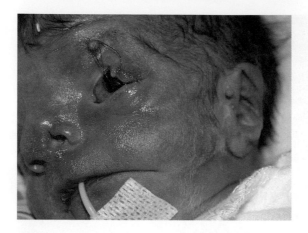

3   Q. Congenital eyelid anomalies – true or false?

a. Epiblepharon is less common than congenital entropion.

b. Epiblepharon usually resolves spontaneously.

c. Congenital lower-lid entropion may be treated by the Hotz procedure.

d. Upper-lid coloboma occurs at the junction of the middle and outer thirds of the eyelid.

e. Lower-lid coloboma occurs in Goldenhar syndrome.

f. Upper-lid coloboma occurs in Treacher Collins syndrome.

A.

a. False. **b.** True. **c.** True. **d.** False – middle and inner third. **e.** False – upper lid (see above). **f.** False – lower lid.

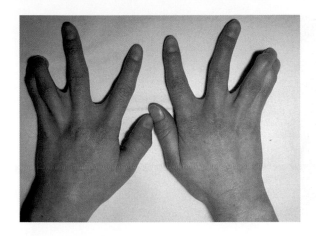

4 Q. Match the syndrome (a–f) with the appropriate description (i–vi).

a. Crouzon syndrome.

b. Apert syndrome.

c. Treacher Collins syndrome.

d. Goldenhar syndrome.

e. Pffeifer syndrome.

f. Halleremann–Streiff–François syndrome.

i. Syndactyly (see above).

ii. Frog-like facies.

iii. Bilateral hypoplasia of the zygoma and mandible.

iv. Broad thumbs and great toes.

v. Membranous cataracts.

vi. Limbal dermoids.

A.

a. & **ii**; b. & **i**; c. & **iii**; d. & **vi**; e. & **iv**; f. & **v**.

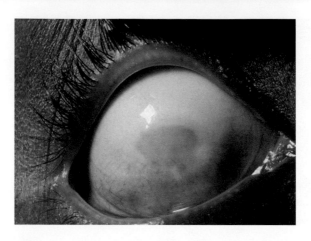

5 **Q. Match the congenital corneal anomaly (a–f) with the appropriate association (i–vi).**

a. Microcornea.

b. Megalocornea.

c. Sclerocornea (see above).

d. Cornea plana.

e. Keratectasia.

f. Posterior keratoconus.

i. Peters anomaly.

ii. K reading of <30D.

iii. Intrauterine keratitis.

iv. Conscriptus.

v. Pigment dispersion syndrome.

vi. AD inheritance

A.

a. & **vi**; b. & **v**; c. & **i**; d. & **ii**; e. & **iii**; f. & **iv**.

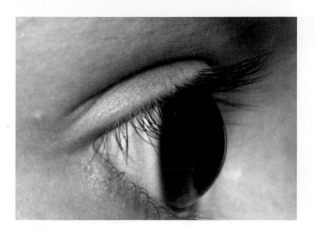

6 Q. Megalocornea – true or false?

a. Inheritance is AD.

b. Iris transillumination is common.

c. Intraocular pressure may become elevated in early adult life.

d. Acute hydrops may occur during the second decade.

e. The corneal diameter is 13 mm or more.

f. Some patients develop renal carcinoma.

A.

a. False – X-linked. **b.** True. **c.** False. **d.** False. **e.** True. **f.** True.

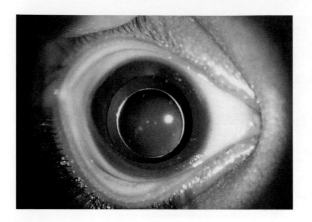

7   Q. Congenital lens anomalies – true or false?

a. Posterior lenticonus is associated with congenital glaucoma.

b. Anterior lenticonus may be associated with retinal flecks.

c. Lentiglobus is usually bilateral.

d. Microsspherophakia (see above) occurs in Weill–Marchesani syndrome.

e. Microphakia is associated with Lowe sydrome.

f. A lens coloboma is not a true coloboma.

A.

a. False. **b.** True – in Alport syndrome. **c.** False. **d.** True. **e.** True.
f. True.

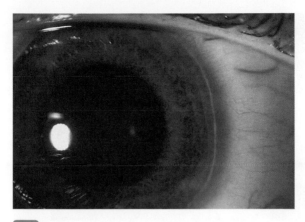

8   **Q. Posterior embryotoxon occurs in the following conditions – true or false?**

a. About 6% of normal eyes.

b. Ehlers–Danlos syndrome.

c. Down syndrome.

d. Axenfeld–Reiger syndrome.

e. Alagille syndrome.

f. Cogan–Reese syndrome.

A.

a. True. **b.** False. **c.** False. **d.** True. **e.** True. **f.** False.

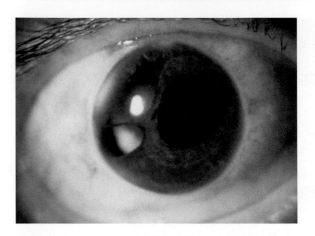

9   Q. Axenfeld–Rieger syndrome – true or false?

a. Involvement is bilateral and symmetrical.

b. Axenfeld anomaly is characterized by attachment of strands of peripheral iris to posterior embryotoxon.

c. Corectopia may occur in Axenfeld anomaly.

d. Ectropion uvea may occur in Rieger anomaly.

e. All patients with Rieger anomaly eventually develop glaucoma.

f. Congenital heart defects are common in Rieger syndrome.

A.

a. False – may be asymmetrical. **b.** True. **c.** False. **d.** True.
e. False – 50%. **f.** False.

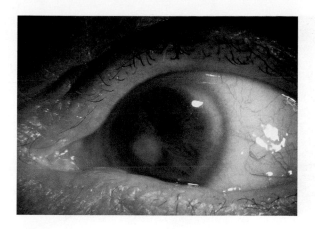

10 Q. Peters anomaly – answer the following.

a. What percentage of cases is bilateral?

b. What is the mode of inheritance?

c. What is the most obvious abnormality?

d. What is the most useful special investigation?

e. What is the incidence of glaucoma?

f. What is the pathogenesis of glaucoma?

A.

a. 80%. b. Most are sporadic. c. Corneal opacity. d. High-frequency ultrasonography (ultrasonic biomicroscopy). e. 50%. f. Incomplete development of the trabecular meshwork and Schlemm canal.

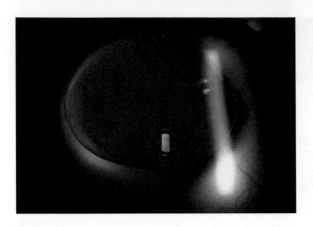

11   Q. Aniridia – true or false?

a. It occurs as a result of abnormal neuroectodermal development secondary to a mutation in the PAX6 gene linked to 11p13.

b. AN-1 is AD and accounts for 66% of cases and has no systemic implications.

c. AN-2 (Miller syndrome) is AR and is associated with cerebellar ataxia.

d. AN-3 (Gillespie syndrome) is sporadic and carries a 30% risk of Wilm tumour.

e. Limbal stem-cell deficiency is common.

f. Glaucoma often presents with buphthalmos.

A.

a. True. **b.** True. **c.** False – sporadic and is not associated with cerebellar ataxia. **d.** False – applies to Miller syndrome. **e.** True. **f.** False.

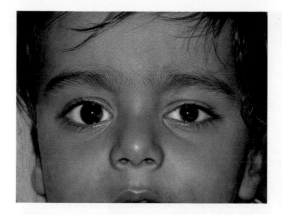

12 Q. Anomalies of globe size – true or false?

a. Microphthalmos (see above) is defined as a total axial length at least two standard deviations below age-similar controls.
b. Complex microphthalmos is often associated with cataract.
c. Microphthalmos with cyst is usually an isolated sporadic condition.
d. Posterior microphthalmos is often associated with retinal detachment.
e. Simple anophthalmos may be associated with absence of extraocular muscles.
f. Nanophthalmos may be associated with uveal effusion.

A.

a. True. **b.** False. **c.** False. **d.** False. **e.** True. **f.** True.

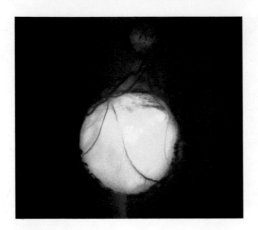

13 Q. Fundus anomalies – answer the following.

a. What is a coloboma?

b. What is the most common mode of inheritance of a chorioretinal coloboma (see above)?

c. What acquired vision-threatening complication may develop in eyes with chorioretinal colobomas?

d. What are ocular associations of eyes with extensive myelinated nerve fibres?

e. What is the mode of inheritance of Aicardi syndrome?

f. What is the characteristic fundus finding in Aicardi syndrome?

A.

a. Absence of part of an ocular structure as a result of incomplete closure of the embryonic fissure. **b.** Usually sporadic. **c.** Retinal breaks that may lead to retinal detachment. **d.** High myopia, anisometropia and amblyopia. **e.** X-linked dominant – it is lethal *in-utero* for males. **f.** Bilateral, multiple depigmented 'chorioretinal lacunae' clustered around the disc.

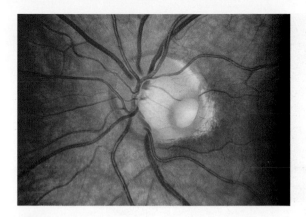

14 Q. Optic disc anomalies – true or false?

a. Tilted discs may be associated with bilateral supero-nasal visual field defects.

b. Eyes with tilted discs are frequently hypermetropic.

c. Serous retinal detachment occurs in 45% of eyes with non-central optic disc pits (see above).

d. The majority of serous retinal detachments in eyes with optic disc pits resolve spontaneously.

e. Patients with optic disc coloboma may have heart defects.

f. Patients with morning glory anomaly may have frontonasal dysplasia.

A.

a. False – supero-temporal. **b.** False – myopic. **c.** True. **d.** False. **e.** True – in 'CHARGE' syndrome. **f.** True.

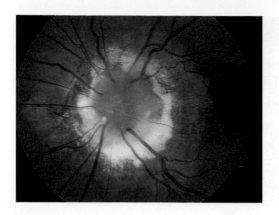

15 Q. The following congenital disc anomalies may be associated with choroidal neovascularization – true or false?

a. Optic disc coloboma.

b. Optic disc pit.

c. Optic disc drusen

d. Tilted disc.

e. Morning glory anomaly (see above).

f. Optic disc hypoplasia.

A.

a. True. b. False. c. True. d. True. e. True. f. False.

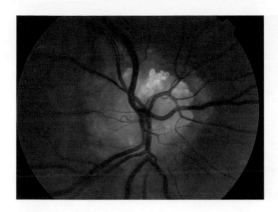

16 Q. Optic disc drusen – answer the following.

a. What is the composition of optic disc drusen?

b. What vascular anomalies are seen in eyes with optic disc drusen?

c. What are fundus associations of optic disc drusen?

d. What systemic syndromic condition is associated with optic disc drusen?

e. What are the findings on fluorescein angiography of exposed optic disc drusen?

f. What is the most readily available investigation for detecting optic disc drusen?

A.

a. Hyaline-like calcific material within the substance of the optic nerve head. **b.** Anomalous vascular patterns are early branching, increased number of major retinal vessels and vascular tortuosity. **c.** Retinitis pigmentosa and angioid streaks. **d.** Allagille syndrome. **e.** Exposed drusen shows the phenomenon of autofluorescence prior to dye injection and then progressive hyperfluorescence due to staining without leakage. **f.** Ultrasonography.

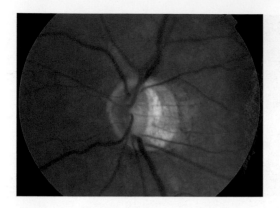

17 Q. Optic nerve hypoplasia – true or false?

a. It is characterized by a diminished number of nerve fibres.
b. It usually occurs as an isolated anomaly in an otherwise normal eye.
c. In mild unilateral cases visual acuity may be improved by patching of the normal eye.
d. In severe cases visual acuity may be no light perception.
e. The retinal blood vessels are usually attenuated.
f. 10% of patients show absence of the septum pellucidum.

A.

a. True. b. True. c. True. d. True. e. False – normal or slightly tortuous.
f. True.

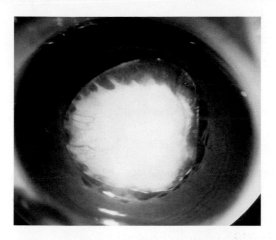

18 Q. Vitreoretinal anomalies – true or false?

a. Persistent hyaloid artery may be associated with a Mittendorf dot.

b. Persistent anterior fetal vasculature (see above) is an important cause of bilateral congenital leukocoria.

c. Eyes with persistent anterior fetal vasculature are usually microphthalmic.

d. Eyes with persistent posterior fetal vasculature have elongated ciliary processes.

e. Patients with Norrie disease usually become blind in early childhood.

f. Patients with incontinentia pigmenti have characteristic cutaneous lesions.

A.

a. True. **b.** False – unilateral **c.** True. **d.** False – persistent anterior fetal vasculature. **e.** False – blind at birth or in early infancy. **f.** True.

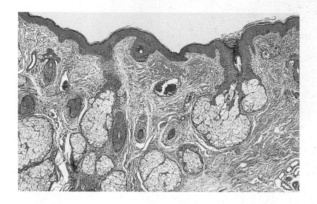

1 **Q. What are the layers of the skin from superficial to deep?**

A.

a. Epidermis consisting of the following layers: i. keratin (horny) layer is very thin and consists of flat, dead cells devoid of nuclei; ii. granular cell layer consists of one or two layers of diamond-shaped or flattened cells containing keratohyaline granules; iii. squamous cell layer is approximately five cells in thickness; iv. basal cell layer comprises a single row of columnar-shaped cells that give rise to more superficial cells. **b.** Dermis containing blood vessels, lymphatics and skin appendages.

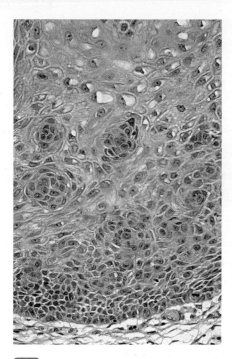

2 **Q. Define.**

a. Hyperkeratosis.
b. Acanthosis.
c. Dyskeratosis.
d. Parakeratosis.
e. Dysplasia.

A.

a. Increase in thickness of the keratin layer and appears clinically as white flaky skin. **b.** Thickening of the squamous cell layer. **c.** Keratinization other than on the surface. **d.** Retention of nuclei into the keratin layer. **e.** Alteration of size, morphology and organization of cellular components (see above).

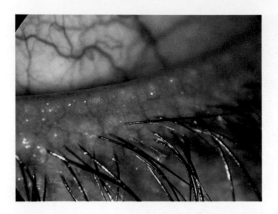

3 Q. Lid margin anatomy – true or false?

a. The mucocutaneous junction corresponds to the grey line.

b. Sebaceous glands are located in the caruncle and within eyebrow hairs.

c. Meibomian glands are modified sebaceous glands in the tarsal plate.

d. Glands of Moll are modified eccrine glands which open into a lash follicle.

e. Glands of Zeis are modified sebaceous glands that are associated with lash follicles.

f. Meibomian glands are more numerous in the lower lid.

A.

a. False. **b.** True. **c.** True. **d.** False – apocrine glands. **e.** True. **f.** False.

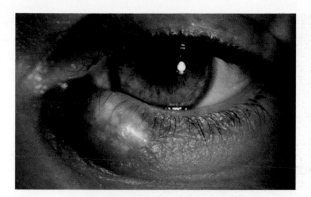

4   Q. Chalazion (meibomian cyst) – true or false?

a. If secondarily infected with *Staphylococcus aureus* it is referred to as external hordeolum.

b. It may disappear spontaneously.

c. It is more common in patients with acne vulgaris.

d. It may present with blurred vision due to astigmatism.

e. Squamous cell carcinoma may mimic 'recurrent' chalazion.

f. Histology shows a lipogranulomatous inflammatory reaction.

A.

a. False – internal hordeolum. **b.** True. **c.** False – acne rosacea. **d.** True.
e. False – meibomian gland carcinoma. **f.** True.

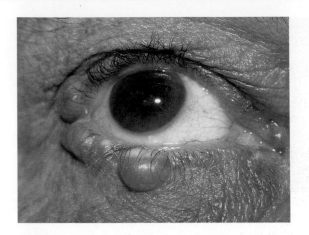

5   Q. Cysts – true or false?

a. A cyst of Moll contains clear fluid.

b. A cyst of Moll may respond to steroid injection.

c. A cyst of Zeis contains sebaceous material.

d. A cyst of Zeis often becomes secondarily infected.

e. A cyst of Zeis typically occurs on the upper eyelid.

f. Sebaceous cysts are often located at the medial canthus.

A.

a. True (see above). **b.** False. **c.** True. **d.** False. **e.** False. **f.** True.

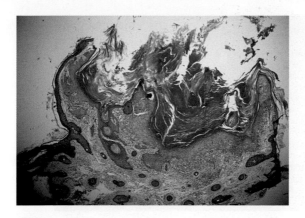

6   **Q. Match the lesion (a–f) with the histological features (i–vi).**

a. Squamous papilloma.

i. Lipid-laden histiocytes within the dermis.

b. Xanthelasma.

ii. Cavity containing keratin lined by keratinized stratified squamous epithelium.

c. Epidermoid cyst.

iii. Elevated expansion of the epidermis by a proliferation of basal cells associated with horn cysts and pseudo-horn cysts.

d. Basal cell papilloma.

iv. Finger-like projections of fibrovascular connective tissue covered by irregular acanthotic and hyperkeratotic squamous epithelium.

e. Actinic keratosis.

v. Keratin-filled crater with irregular thickened epidermis surrounded by acanthotic squamous epithelium (see above).

f. Keratoacanthoma.

vi. Irregular dysplastic epidermis with hyperkeratosis and parakeratosis.

A.

a. & **iv**; **b.** & **i**; **c.** & **ii**; **d.** & **iii**; **e.** & **vi**; **f.** & **v**.

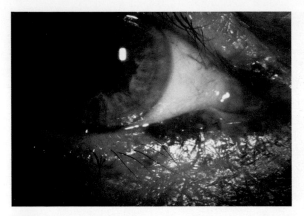

7   Q. What have these in common?

a. Bowen disease.

b. Hutchinson freckle (see above).

c. Actinic keratosis.

d. Xeroderma pigmentosum.

A.

They are all premalignant conditions.

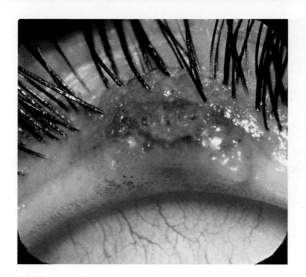

8 Q. Naevus – answer the following.

a. What is a naevus (see above)?
b. How are naevi classified histologically?
c. Which type carries no risk for malignant transformation?
d. What are the indications for surgical excision?

A.

a. A benign lesion composed of naevus cells (naevocytes). **b.** According to the location of naevus cells within the skin: into junctional, compound and intradermal. **c.** Intradermal. **d.** Cosmetic reasons and concern regarding possible malignancy.

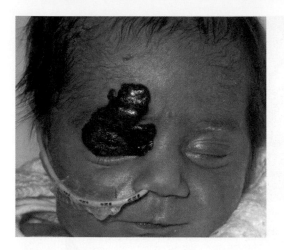

9

Q. Strawberry naevus (capillary haemangioma) – true or false?

a. It is more common in boys than girls.

b. Presents shortly after birth.

c. Blanches with pressure.

d. Spontaneous regression usually occurs by the age of 3 years.

e. Treatment may involve both steroid injections and systemic steroid administration.

f. May be associated with orbital extension.

A.

a. False. **b.** True. **c.** True. **d.** False – 7 years. **e.** True. **f.** True.

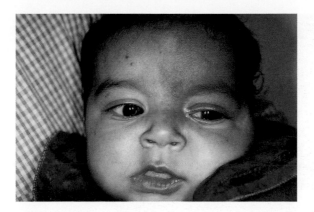

10 Q. Port wine stain (naevus flammeus) – true or false?

a. With time the overlying skin becomes thin and atrophic.

b. It blanches with pressure.

c. It may be associated with ipsilateral glaucoma.

d. It may be associated with ipsilateral circumscribed choroidal haemangioma.

e. Most cases are not associated with Sturge–Weber syndrome.

f. Treatment involves surgical excision.

A.

a. False – hypertrophied and coarse. **b.** False. **c.** True. **d.** False – diffuse choroidal haemangioma. **e.** True. **f.** False.

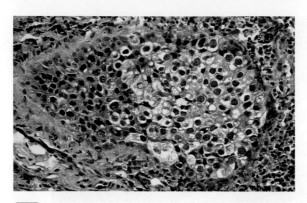

11 **Q. Match the malignant tumour (a–d) with the appropriate histological feature (i–iv).**

a. Kaposi sarcoma.

b. Melanoma.

c. Basal cell carcinoma.

d. Sebaceous carcinoma.

i. Downward proliferation of basal cells.

ii. Large atypical melanocytes within the dermis.

iii. Proliferating spindle cells, vascular channels and inflammatory cells within the dermis.

iv. Lobules of cells with pale foamy vacuolated cytoplasm and large hyperchromatic nuclei (see above).

A.

a. & **iii**; **b.** & **ii**; **c.** & **i**; **d.** & **iv**.

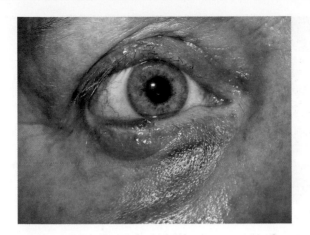

12 Q. Basal cell carcinoma – true or false?

a. Is the most prevalent malignant eyelid tumour.

b. The sclerosing type (see above) is most common.

c. Most frequently arises from the lower lid.

d. Metastatic spread to regional lymph nodes is common at presentation.

e. It may exhibit pagetoid spread.

f. It should never be treated by radiotherapy.

A.

a. True. **b.** False – ulcerative. **c.** True. **d.** False. **e.** False – sebaceous carcinoma. **f.** False.

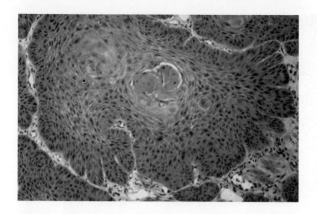

13   Q. Squamous cell carcinoma – true or false?

a. Histology of poorly differentiated tumours may show keratin 'pearls'.

b. It is the most aggressive of eyelid malignancy.

c. Patients with AIDS are at increased risk.

d. Regional lymph node involvement is very rare.

e. It may exhibit perineural spread to the intracranial cavity.

f. It is usually be treated by radiotherapy.

A.

a. False – well-differentiated tumours (see above). **b.** False – more aggressive are Merkel cell carcinoma, sebaceous cell carcinoma and melanoma. **c.** True. **d.** False – 20% of cases. **e.** True. **f.** False.

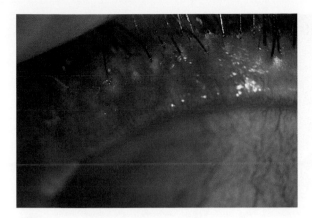

14 Q. Malignant tumours – true or false?

a. Sebaceous gland carcinoma has a predilection for the upper lid.

b. Sebaceous gland carcinoma may mimic benign conditions such as blepharitis.

c. Sebaceous gland carcinoma has 5% 5-year mortality.

d. Most melanomas arise from Hutchinson freckle.

e. Melanomas are clinically non-pigmented in 50% of cases.

f. Patients with Merkel cell carcinoma frequently show metastatic spread at presentation.

A.

a. True. **b.** True (see above). **c.** False – 30%. **d.** False. **e.** True. **f.** True.

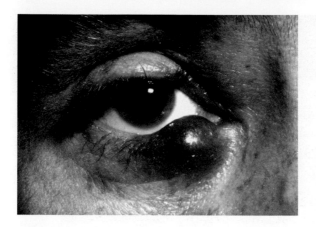

15   Q. Treatment of malignant tumours – true or false?

a. Mohs' technique is frequently associated with removal of excessive healthy tissue.

b. The recurrence rates of basal cell carcinoma treated by excision and radiotherapy are the same.

c. Kaposi sarcoma (see above) is very sensitive to radiotherapy.

d. Cryotherapy may damage the canalicular system.

e. Medial canthal basal cell carcinoma may be treated by radiotherapy.

f. Sclerosing basal cell carcinoma must not be treated by radiotherapy.

A.

a. False. **b.** False – radiotherapy is higher. **c.** True. **d.** False. **e.** False.
f. True.

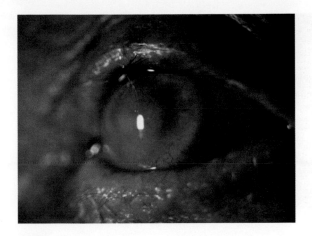

16 Q. Trichiasis – true or false?

a. It may cause pannus.

b. Pseudo-trichiasis does not cause punctate epithelial erosions.

c. May be difficult to differentiate from distichiasis.

d. Treatment with cryotherapy may adversely affect the precorneal tear film.

e. Electrolysis has the advantage of preventing recurrence.

f. May be caused by herpes zoster ophthalmicus.

A.

a. True. **b.** False. **c.** False. **d.** True. **e.** False. **f.** True (see above).

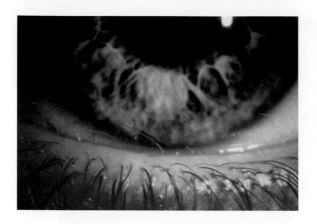

17 Q. Congenital distichiasis – true or false?

a. Inheritance is AD.

b. The aberrant lashes are thicker and longer than normal lashes.

c. Symptoms usually occur in infancy.

d. May be associated with lymphoedema of the legs.

e. Treatment of lower-lid distichiasis involves lamellar eyelid division and cryotherapy.

f. The aberrant lashes emerge in front of meibomian gland orifices.

A.

a. True. **b.** False – thinner and shorter (see above). **c.** False – may not occur until the age of 5 years. **d.** True. **e.** False – upper lid distichiasis. **f.** False – emerge at or slightly behind meibomian gland orifices.

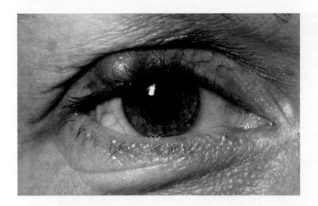

18 Q. Stye – true or false?

a. Is synonymous with external hordeolum.

b. Is frequently associated with seborrhoeic blepharitis.

c. Is an acute staphylococcal infection of a gland of Moll.

d. May require incision and curettage.

e. May progress to chalazion.

f. Is common in children.

A.

a. True. **b.** False – staphylococcal blepharitis. **c.** False. **d.** False. **e.** False.
f. True.

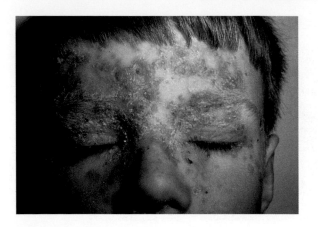

19   Q. Infections – true or false?

a. Impetigo most frequently affects elderly individuals.

b. Treatment of impetigo with oral erythromycin may be appropriate.

c. Erysipelas is typically produces golden-yellow crusts.

d. Erysipelas is usually associated with minor skin trauma.

e. Necrotizing fasciitis is usually caused by *Staphylococcus aureus*.

f. Treatment of necrotizing fasciitis is with oral phenoxymethylpenicillin.

A.

a. False – children. **b.** True. **c.** False – impetigo (see above). **d.** True.

e. False – *Streptococcus pyogenes*. **f.** False – intravenous benzylpenicillin.

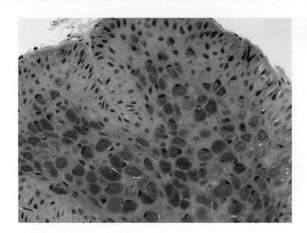

20 Q. Molluscum contagiosum – answer the following.

a. What is the name of the intracytoplasmic inclusion bodies seen on histology?
b. Are the inclusion bodies larger near the surface of the lesion or deeper down?
c. What is the nature of the virus?
d. What is the peak incidence of infection?
e. What ocular complications may occur in patients with a lesion on the lid margin?
f. What is the distribution of facial molluscum lesions in AIDS?

A.

a. Henderson–Patterson. **b.** Larger deeper down (see above). **c.** Human specific double stranded DNA poxvirus. **d.** Between 2 and 4 years.
e. Ipsilateral chronic follicular conjunctivitis. **f.** Chinstrap distribution.

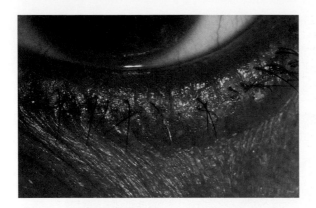

21 **Q. Chronic marginal blepharitis – true or false?**

a. Symptoms provide a reliable clue as to the type of blepharitis.

b. Anterior blepharitis is frequently associated with acne rosacea.

c. In staphylococcal blepharitis the scales are located anywhere on the lid margin.

d. Froth on the lid margin may be seen in posterior blepharitis.

e. Treatment with minocycline may cause skin pigmentation.

f. With appropriate treatment a permanent cure is usually possible.

A.

a. False. **b.** False – posterior blepharitis. **c.** False – around the base of the lashes (collarettes, see above). **d.** True. **e.** True. **f.** False.

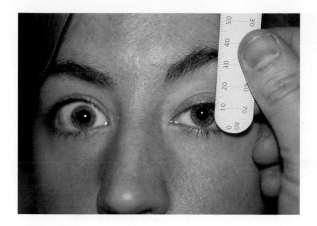

22 Q. Examination of the upper eyelid – true or false?

a. The normal margin–reflex distance is 3.5 mm.

b. The palpebral fissure height (see above) is greater in females than in males.

c. Mild ptosis measures 3 mm or less.

d. Levator function of 4 mm or less is considered poor.

e. A high upper-lid crease is suggestive of an aponeurotic defect.

f. Pretarsal show is the distance between the lid margin and the skin fold with the eyes in the primary position.

A.

a. False – 4–4.5 mm. **b.** True. **c.** False – up to 2 mm. **d.** True. **e.** True.
f. True.

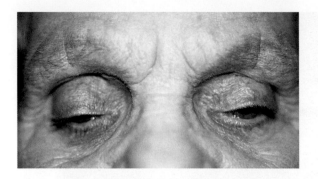

23   Q. The following statements are correctly associated – true or false?

a. Congenital ptosis and defective elevation of the eye.

b. Aponeurotic ptosis (see above) and good levator function.

c. 4 mm of ptosis in Horner syndrome.

d. Lid elevation on moving the jaw in aberrant regeneration of the third nerve.

e. Pseudoptosis and ipsilateral hypertropia.

f. Myasthenic ptosis and Cogan twitch sign.

A.

a. True. **b.** True. **c.** False. **d.** False. **e.** False – hypotropia. **f.** True.

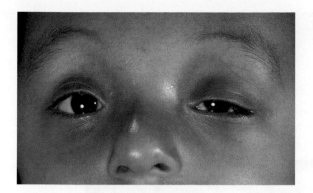

24 Q. Simple congenital ptosis – true or false?

a. The majority of cases are hereditary.

b. The upper-lid crease is frequently absent.

c. It is invariably unilateral.

d. In downgaze the ptotic lid is higher than the normal.

e. Refractive errors are common.

f. Most cases require levator resection.

A.

a. False. **b.** True (see above). **c.** False. **d.** True. **e.** True. **f.** True.

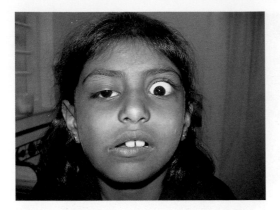

25 Q. Marcus Gunn jaw-winking syndrome – true or false?

a. Comprises about 5% of all cases of congenital ptosis.

b. Most cases are unilateral.

c. Retraction of the ptotic lid occurs on jaw movement to the ipsilateral side.

d. It usually improves with age.

e. Bilateral surgery may be required.

f. It may be associated with Down syndrome.

A.

a. True. **b.** True. **c.** False – contralateral side (see above). **d.** False.
e. True. **f.** False.

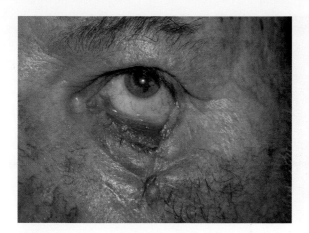

26   Q. Ectropion – true or false?

a. Involutional ectropion is principally caused by disinsertion of the lower-lid retractors.

b. Mild involutional ectropion may be treated by the Weis procedure.

c. Horizontal lid laxity in involutional ectropion is demonstrated by pushing the lower lid laterally and observing the position of the inferior punctum.

d. Cicatricial ectropion (see above) may require treatment with transposition flaps.

e. Paralytic ectropion may be associated with brow ptosis.

f. Paralytic ectropion may be treated by lower-lid shortening.

A.

a. False. **b.** False – entropion. **c.** False – demonstrates medial canthal tendon laxity. **d.** True. **e.** True. **f.** False.

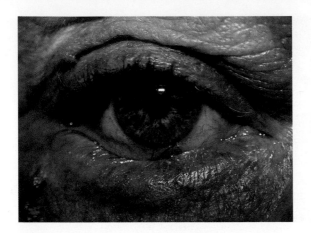

27   Q. Involutional entropion – true or false?

a. May cause pseudo-trichiasis.

b. Is associated with over-riding of the preseptal by the pretarsal orbicularis.

c. Horizontal lid laxity is caused by disinsertion of the lower-lid retractors.

d. Jones procedure tightens the lower-lid retractors.

e. Temporary treatment may involve botulinum toxin injection.

f. Transverse everting sutures may result in permanent cure.

A.

a. True (see above). **b.** False – over-riding of the pretarsal by the preseptal orbicularis. **c.** False – disinsertion of lower-lid retractors causes vertical lid instability. **d.** True. **e.** True. **f.** False – temporary.

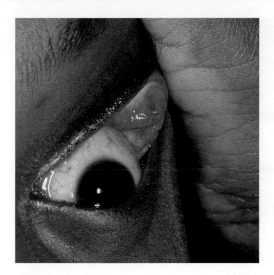

28 Q. Miscellaneous eyelid conditions – true or false?

a. Blepharochalasis typically presents in middle age.

b. Blepharochalasis is characterized by transient pitting eyelid oedema.

c. Dermatochalasis may cause a pseudo-ptosis.

d. Floppy eyelid syndrome (see above) typically affects obese men.

e. Floppy eyelid syndrome may cause chronic follicular conjunctivitis.

f. In the eyelid imbrication syndrome, the upper lid overlaps the lower.

A.

a. False – at about puberty. **b.** False – non-pitting. **c.** True. **d.** True.
e. False – papillary. **f.** True.

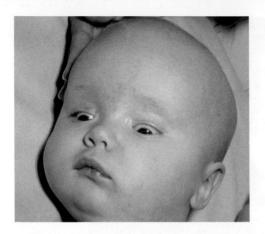

29   Q. What have these conditions in common?

a. Duane syndrome.

b. Parinaud syndrome.

c. Hydrocephalus (see above).

d. Aberrant third nerve regeneration.

e. Marcus Gunn jaw-winking.

f. Parkinson's disease.

A.

They are all associated with lid retraction.

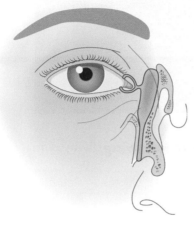

1 Q. Anatomy – true or false?

a. The lacrimal bone and the frontal process of the maxilla separate the lacrimal sac from the superior meatus of the nasal cavity.

b. 50% of tears drain through the upper canaliculus.

c. The lacrimal sac lies between the anterior and posterior lacrimal crests.

d. The nasolacrimal duct opens lateral to and below the inferior meatus.

e. The opening of the nasolacrimal duct is covered by the valve of Rosenmüller.

f. The nasolacrimal duct passes downwards, laterally and posteriorly.

A.

a. False – middle meatus. **b.** False – 30%. **c.** True. **d.** True. **e.** False – Hasner. **f.** True.

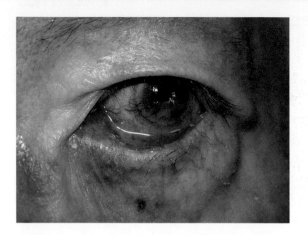

2   **Q. Define the following.**

a. Centurion syndrome.

b. Conjunctivochalasis.

c. Epiphora.

d. Secondary punctal stenosis.

e. Pars lacrimalis.

f. Lacrimation.

A.

a. Anterior malposition of the medial part of the lid with displacement
of the puncta out of the lacus lacrimalis. **b.** Redundant fold of conjunctiva.
c. A sign of overflow of tears. **d.** Caused by medial ectropion (see above).
e. The medial one-sixth non-lash bearing part of the lid. **f.** Hypersecretion
of tears.

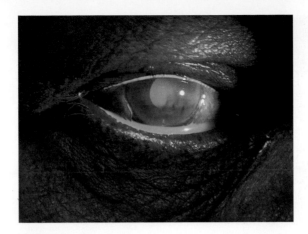

3   Q. Investigations – true or false?

a. Negative primary Jones test is indicative of lacrimal pump failure.

b. Positive primary Jones test indicates patency of the lacrimal system.

c. Hard stop is indicative of a stone in the lacrimal sac.

d. Soft stop excludes complete obstruction of the lacrimal system.

e. Distension of the lacrimal sac on syringing is indicative of total obstruction of the nasolacrimal sac.

f. A normal fluorescein disappearance test (see above) shows little or no residual dye after 3 minutes.

A.

a. True. **b.** True. **c.** False. **d.** False. **e.** True. **f.** True.

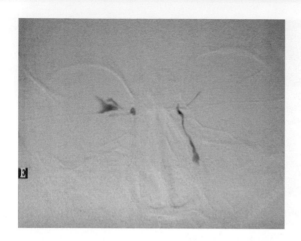

4   Q. Special investigations – true or false?

a. Contrast dacryocystography (see above) is most useful in patients with mucoceles.

b. Contrast dacryocystography should not be performed in patients with acute dacryocystitis.

c. Contrast dacryocystography provides more detailed anatomical visualization than nuclear lacrimal scintigraphy.

d. Nuclear lacrimal scintigraphy is more physiological than contrast dacryocystography.

e. Nuclear lacrimal scintigraphy utilizes radionuclide strontium 88.

f. In nuclear lacrimal scintigraphy images are recorded over 20 minutes.

A.

a. False. **b.** True. **c.** True. **d.** True. **e.** False – technetium 99. **f.** True.

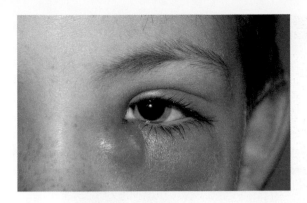

5   Q. True or false?

a. Secondary punctal stenosis may be treated by lower-lid tightening.

b. Naso-orbital trauma is the most common cause of acquired nasolacrimal duct obstruction.

c. Dacryolithiasis may present with recurrent acute dacryocystitis.

d. Chronic canaliculitis is frequently secondary to nasolacrimal duct obstruction.

e. Dacryocystitis is usually secondary to common canalicular obstruction.

f. Acute dacryocystitis (see above) may be treated by incision and drainage in certain circumstances.

A.

a. True. **b.** False – most are idiopathic. **c.** True. **d.** False. **e.** False – nasolacrimal duct obstruction. **f.** True.

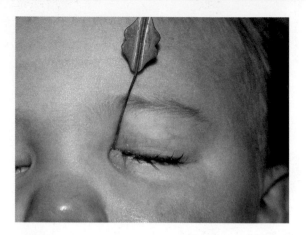

6   Q. True or false?

a. Most cases of congenital nasolacrimal duct obstruction require probing (see above).

b. Chronic canaliculitis can usually be cured medically.

c. Dacryocystorhinostomy is indicated for obstruction beyond the medial opening of the common canaliculus.

d. Balloon dacryocystoplasty may be used in adults with partial nasolacrimal duct obstruction.

e. A Lester Jones tube may be considered in lacrimal pump failure.

f. The 'sump syndrome' is a cause of failure of dacryocystorhinostomy.

A.

a. False – 95% clear spontaneously by 12 months of age. **b.** False – most require canaliculotomy. **c.** True. **d.** True. **e.** True. **f.** True.

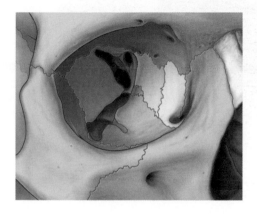

1 Q. Orbital anatomy – complete the following sentences.

a. The roof consists of two bones: lesser wing of the sphenoid and ... .
b. The lateral wall also consists of two bones: greater wing of the sphenoid and ... .
c. The floor consists of three bones: zygomatic, maxillary and ... .
d. The medial wall consists of four bones: maxillary, lacrimal, ethmoid and ... .
e. The superior portion of the superior orbital fissure contains the lacrimal, frontal and trochlear nerves, and ... .
f. The inferior portion contains the superior and inferior divisions of the oculomotor nerve, the abducens, the nasociliary and ... .

A.

a. Orbital plate of the frontal. **b.** Zygomatic. **c.** Palatine. **d.** Sphenoid.
e. Superior ophthalmic vein. **f.** Sympathetic fibres.

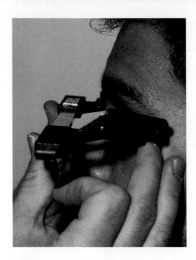

2   Q. Proptosis – true or false?

a. Cavernous haemangioma usually gives rise to eccentric proptosis.

b. Optic nerve tumours give rise to axial proptosis.

c. Exophthalmometer (see above) readings greater than 20 mm are indicative of proptosis.

d. Difference in exophthalmometer readings between the two eyes of 3 mm or more is suspicious regardless of the absolute reading.

e. Proptosis of 24 would be considered mild.

f. Proptosis of 29 would be considered severe.

A.

a. False – axial. **b.** True. **c.** True. **d.** False – 2 mm. **e.** False – 21–23 mm.
f. True.

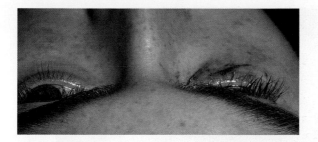

3 Q. What have the following conditions in common?

a. Leber amaurosis.

b. Breast carcinoma.

c. Idiopathic orbital inflammatory disease.

d. Scleroderma.

e. Orbital varices.

f. Blow-out fracture of the orbital floor.

A.

They may all be associated with enophthalmos (see above).

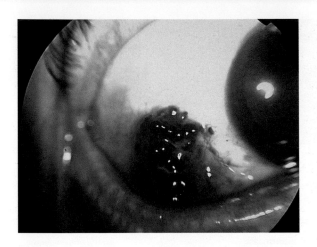

4   Q. Answer the following.

a. How may an optic nerve sheath meningioma cause diplopia?
b. What is the purpose of forced duction testing?
c. What constitutes a positive response in the differential intraocular pressure test?
d. Which conditions may exacerbate or induce proptosis on the Valsalva manoeuvre?
e. What may cause pulsatile proptosis without a bruit?
f. What may cause pulsatile proptosis with a bruit?

A.

a. By splinting the optic nerve. **b.** To differentiate a restrictive from a neurological motility defect. **c.** An increase of intraocular pressure of 6 mm or more on upgaze. **d.** Orbital venous anomalies (see above) or capillary orbital haemangioma. **e.** Defect in the orbital roof that transmits pulsation from the brain by cerebrospinal fluid. **f.** Arteriovenous communication such as a carotid-cavernous fistula.

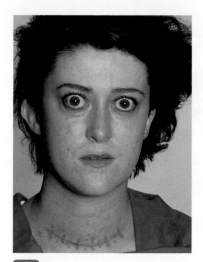

5 **Q. Thyroid eye disease and hyperthyroidism – true or false?**

a. Hyperthyroidism typically presents in the fourth to fifth decades.

b. Hyperthyroidism is more common in females than males.

c. About 15% of patients with hyperthyroidism develop thyroid eye disease.

d. The major risk factor for thyroid eye disease is smoking.

e. Thyroid eye disease may be improved by taking radioactive iodine to treat hyperthyroidism.

f. Thyroid eye disease is five times more common in females than males.

A.

a. False – third to fourth decades. **b.** True. **c.** False – 25–50%. **d.** True. **e.** False. **f.** True.

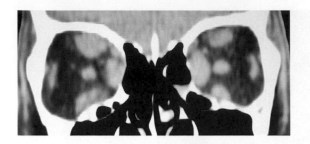

6   Q. Thyroid eye disease – true or false?

a. The congestive phase tends to remit within 3 years.

b. It may affect children.

c. Epibulbar hyperaemia is a sensitive indicator of inflammatory activity.

d. The most commonly involved muscle is the medial rectus.

e. Extraocular muscle enlargement (see above) and orbital tissues infiltration is associated with increased accumulation of mucopolysaccharides.

f. Asymmetrical involvement is common.

A.

a. True. **b.** True. **c.** True. **d.** False – inferior rectus. **e.** False – glycansaminoglycans not mucopolysaccharides. **f.** True.

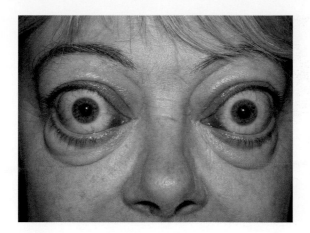

7 Q. Lid retraction in thyroid eye disease – true or false?

a. It is suspected when the lid margin is above the superior limbus (see above).

b. It occurs in about 50% of patients with hyperthyroidism.

c. Lid retraction in downgaze is caused by fibrotic contracture of the levator associated with adhesions with the overlying orbital tissues.

d. Kocher sign describes lid retraction in the primary position.

e. von Graefe sign signifies retarded descent on the upper lid on downgaze.

f. It may be alleviated by botulinum toxin injection.

A.
a. False – level with the superior limbus. **b.** True. **c.** True. **d.** False – frightened appearance on attentive gaze. **e.** True. **f.** True.

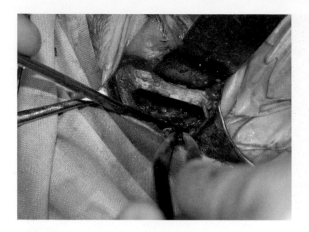

8   Q. Treatment of thyroid eye disease – answer the following.

a. What is the usual initial dose of oral steroids?

b. How is intravenous methylprednisolone administered?

c. How long does it take for radiotherapy to take effect?

d. How much retroplacement of proptosis is achieved by a three-wall decompression (see above)?

e. What are the main indications for strabismus surgery?

f. What does strabismus surgery usually involve?

A.

a. Prednisolone 60–80 mg/day. **b.** 0.5 g in 200 ml isotonic saline solution over 30 minutes. **c.** 6 weeks. **d.** 6–10 mm. **e.** Diplopia in the primary or reading position of gaze provided the disease is quiescent and the angle of deviation has been stable for at least 6 months. **f.** Recession of the fibrotic muscle, preferably using adjustable sutures.

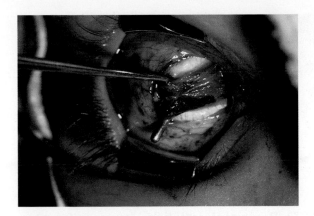

9   Q. The correct sequence of surgery for thyroid eye disease is – true or false?

a. Orbit, lids, strabismus (see above).

b. Orbit, strabismus, lids.

c. Lids, strabismus, orbit.

d. Lids, orbit, strabismus.

e. Strabismus, orbit, lids.

f. Strabismus, lids, orbit.

A.

a. False. **b.** True. **c.** False. **d.** False. **e.** False. **f.** False.

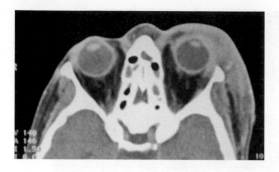

10   Q. Preseptal cellulitis – true or false?

a. It is an infection of the subcutaneous tissues anterior to the orbital septum.

b. It may be caused by dacryocystitis.

c. *Haemophilus influenzae* is a common pathogen.

d. It never progresses to orbital cellulitis.

e. Mild proptosis is common.

f. Treatment always requires hospital admission.

A.

a. True (see above). **b.** True. **c.** False – *Staphylococcus aureus* and *Streptococcus pyogenes*. **d.** False. **e.** False. **f.** False.

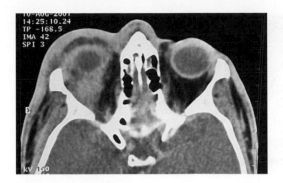

11 Q. Bacterial orbital cellulitis – answer the following.

a. Define bacterial orbital cellulitis.

b. At what age does it usually present?

c. What are the most common causative pathogens?

d. What is the most common primary source of the infection?

e. What are the ocular complications?

f. What is the antimicrobial treatment?

A.

a. Life-threatening infection of the soft tissues behind the orbital septum (see above). **b.** In childhood. **c.** *Streptococcus pneumoniae, Staphylococcus aureus, Streptococcus pyogenes* and *Haemophilus influenzae.* **d.** Ethmoidal sinusitis. **e.** Exposure keratopathy, raised intraocular pressure, occlusion of the central retinal artery or vein, endophthalmitis and optic neuropathy. **f.** Intramuscular ceftazidine 1 g every 8 hours and oral metronidazole 500 mg every 8 hours.

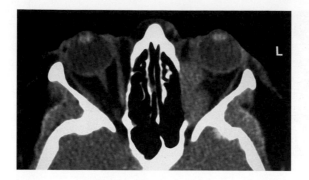

12   Q. Idiopathic orbital inflammatory disease (pseudotumour) – true or false?

a. Histological and clinical features are strongly related.

b. In adults the condition is frequently bilateral.

c. Simultaneous orbital and sinus involvement is common.

d. CT shows ill-defined opacification.

e. Treatment with non-steroidal anti-inflammatory agents is not usually effective.

f. Spontaneous remission may occur after several weeks.

A.

a. False. **b.** False. **c.** False. **d.** True (see above). **e.** False. **f.** True.

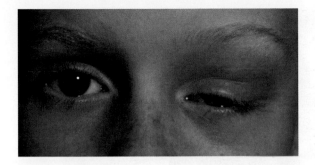

13 Q. Orbital inflammation – true or false?

a. Acute dacryoadenitis (see above) usually does not require treatment.

b. In orbital myositis diplopia occurs away from the field of action of the involved muscle.

c. CT in acute orbital myositis shows diffuse enlargement of the involved muscle.

d. Tolosa–Hunt syndrome is associated with sensory loss along the distribution of the first and second divisions of the trigeminal nerve.

e. Treatment of Tolosa–Hunt is with radiotherapy.

f. Orbital involvement in Wegener granulomatosis is often bilateral.

A.

a. True. **b.** False – into the field of the involved muscle. **c.** False – fusiform enlargement. **d.** True. **e.** False – systemic steroids. **f.** True.

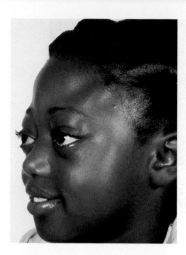

14   Q. The following may involve both orbits – true or false?

a. Non-Hodgkin lymphoma.

b. Metastasis.

c. Acute childhood leukaemia.

d. Tuberculosis.

e. Graves disease.

f. Fungal infection.

A.

a. True. **b.** False. **c.** True (see above). **d.** True. **e.** True. **f.** False.

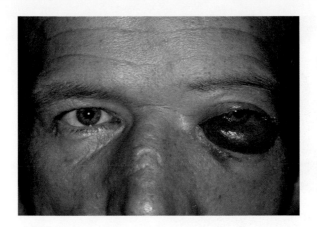

15 Q. Carotid-cavernous fistula – answer the following.

a. How is it classified?

b. What is the most common cause of direct carotid-cavernous fistula?

c. Which individuals are at highest risk of spontaneous carotid-cavernous fistula?

d. What are the signs of anterior segment ischaemia?

e. What is the direction of blood flow in indirect carotid-cavernous fistula?

f. What is interventional radiology?

A.

a. Based on aetiology (spontaneous and traumatic), haemodynamics (high and low flow) and anatomy (direct and indirect). **b.** Trauma is responsible for 75% of cases. **c.** Post-menopausal hypertensive women. **d.** Corneal epithelial oedema, aqueous cells and flare, iris atrophy, cataract and rubeosis iridis. **e.** Arterial blood flows through the meningeal branches of the external or internal carotid arteries indirectly into the cavernous sinus. **f.** Detachable balloon occlusion of the fistula.

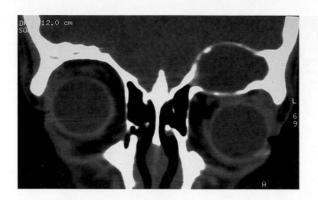

16   Q. Orbital cystic lesions – true or false?

a. Dermoid cyst is a hamartoma.

b. A ruptured superficial dermoid cyst may mimic acute dacryoadenitis.

c. Deep dermoid cysts typically present in infancy.

d. Frontal mucocele may invade the orbit.

e. Posterior encephalocele is characterized by pulsating proptosis and a bruit.

f. Anterior encephalocele may be associated with neurofibromatosis-1.

A.

a. False – choristoma. **b.** True. **c.** False – adolescence or adult life.
d. True (see above). **e.** False – bruit is not present. **f.** False – posterior encephalocele.

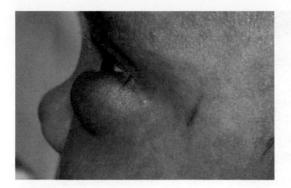

17 Q. Orbital capillary haemangiomas – true or false?

a. It is a hamartoma.

b. Histologically it is composed of varying-sized small vascular channels.

c. Majority are present at birth.

d. Inferior anterior orbit is most commonly involved (see above).

e. Ultrasonography is essential in guiding the appropriate treatment.

f. It is usually well encapsulated and easy to remove.

A.

a. True. **b.** True. **c.** False – 30%. **d.** False – superior anterior. **e.** True. **f.** False.

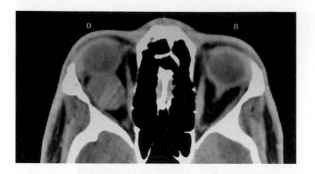

18   Q. Orbital cavernous haemangioma – answer the following.

a. Is it more common in females or males?

b. What is the most common location in the orbit?

c. What does histology show?

d. At what age and how does it present?

e. What is the most important systemic association?

f. What is the treatment?

A.

a. Female preponderance is 70%. **b.** Within the lateral part of the muscle cone just behind the globe (see above). **c.** Endothelial-lined vascular channels of varying size separated by fibrous septae. **d.** In the fourth to fifth decades with slowly progressive unilateral axial proptosis. **e.** It is not associated with systemic conditions. **f.** Surgical excision.

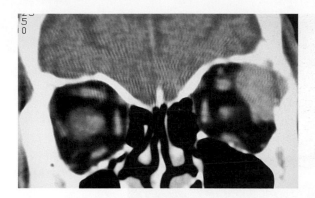

19 Q. Lacrimal gland tumours – true or false?

a. Pleomorphic adenoma (benign mixed-cell tumour) is the most common tumour of the lacrimal gland.

b. Treatment of pleomorphic adenoma involves biopsy followed by surgical excision.

c. CT of pleomorphic adenoma shows bony destruction.

d. Lacrimal gland carcinoma may occur after incomplete excision of pleomorphic adenoma.

e. Lacrimal gland carcinoma may cause choroidal folds.

f. Lacrimal gland carcinoma carries a poor prognosis for life.

A.

a. True. **b.** False – biopsy should be avoided. **c.** False – carcinoma causes bony destruction (see above), adenoma causes indentation. **d.** True.
e. True. **f.** True.

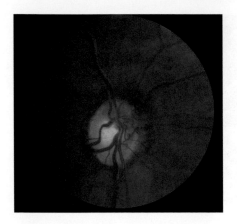

20 **Q. Neural orbital tumours – answer the following.**

a. What systemic condition may be associated with optic nerve glioma?

b. At what age and how does optic glioma present?

c. What are the characteristics of optic nerve glioma on MR?

d. What are the indications for surgical excision of optic nerve glioma?

e. What is the classical triad of optic nerve sheath meningioma?

f. What are the findings of CT optic nerve sheath meningioma?

A.

a. Neurofibromatosis-1 is present in 30% of cases. **b.** First decade of life (median age 6.5 years) with slowly-progressive visual loss visual loss, followed later by proptosis. **c.** MR T1-weighted images are hypo- to isointense; T2-weighted scans are hyperintense. **d.** Large or growing tumours that are confined to the orbit, particularly if vision is poor and proptosis significant. **e.** Visual loss, optic atrophy and opticociliary vessels (see above). **f.** Thickening and calcification of the optic nerve.

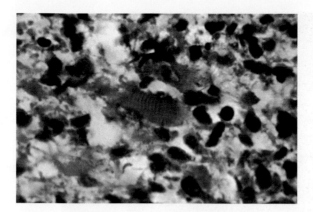

21 Q. Orbital embryonal sarcoma – true or false?

a. It arises from striated muscle.

b. It is the most common orbital malignancy in childhood.

c. It may initially be mistaken for an inflammatory process.

d. The most common location is inferonasal.

e. CT often shows bony destruction.

f. Initial treatment involves surgical excision.

A.

a. False – it arises from undifferentiated mesenchymal cell rests which have the potential to differentiate into striated muscle (see above). **b.** True. **c.** True. **d.** False – superotemporal or retrobulbar. **e.** True. **f.** False – radiotherapy and chemotherapy.

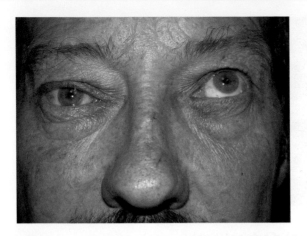

22 **Q. Match the orbital lesion (a–f) with the most appropriate finding (i–vi).**

a. Orbital varices.

b. Optic nerve sheath meningioma.

c. Metastatic carcinoma.

d. Lymphoma.

e. Lymphangioma.

f. Metastatic neuroblastoma.

i. Diplopia in upgaze (see above).

ii. Intermittent proptosis.

iii. Eyelid ecchymosis.

iv. Enophthalmos.

v. Bilateral proptosis.

vi. 'Chocolate cysts'.

A.

a. & **ii**; **b.** & **i**; **c.** & **iv**; **d.** & **v**; **e.** & **vi**; **f.** & **iii**.

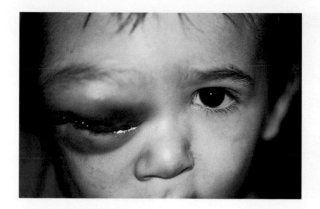

23 **Q. The following present in childhood – true or false?**

a. Lymphangioma.

b. Langerhans cell granulomatosis.

c. Embryonal sarcoma.

d. Plexiform neurofibroma (see above).

e. Cavernous haemangioma.

f. Optic nerve glioma.

A.

a. True. **b.** True. **c.** True. **d.** True. **e.** False. **f.** True.

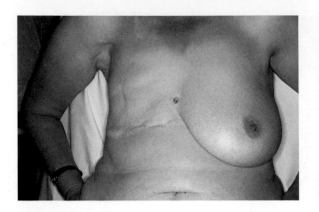

24 **Q. The following primary tumours may metastasize to the orbit – true or false?**

a. Pancreas.

b. Bronchus.

c. Ovary.

d. Neuroblastoma.

e. Breast (see above).

f. Kidney.

A.

a. False. **b.** True. **c.** False. **d.** True. **e.** True. **f.** True.

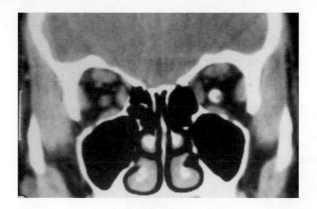

25 Q. The following may show calcification on CT – true or false?

a. Orbital varices.

b. Cavernous haemangioma.

c. Optic nerve sheath meningioma.

d. Retinoblastoma.

e. Lacrimal gland carcinoma.

f. Optic nerve glioma.

A.

a. True. **b.** False. **c.** True (see above). **d.** True. **e.** True. **f.** False.

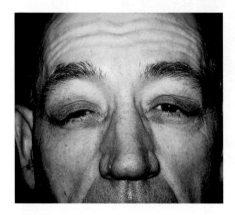

1 Q. Define the following.

a. Keratoconjunctivitis sicca (KCS).

b. Xerophthalmia.

c. Xerosis.

d. Xerostomia.

e. Sjögren syndrome.

f. Mikulicz syndrome.

A.

a. Any eye with some degree of dryness. **b.** Dry eye associated with vitamin A deficiency. **c.** Extreme ocular dryness and keratinization that occurs in eyes with severe conjunctival cicatrization. **d.** Dry mouth.

e. Autoimmune inflammatory disease usually associated with dry eyes.

f. Chronic bilateral hypertrophy of lacrimal (see above) and salivary glands often accompanied by systemic disease such as sarcoidosis and lymphoma.

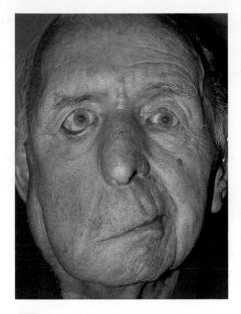

2 Q. Causes of non-Sjögren dry eye – true or false?

a. Sarcoidosis.

b. Riley–Day syndrome.

c. Refractive surgery.

d. Stevens–Johnson syndrome.

e. Facial nerve palsy (see above).

f. Parkinson's disease.

A.

a. True. **b.** True. **c.** True. **d.** True. **e.** False – causes evaporative KCS.
f. True.

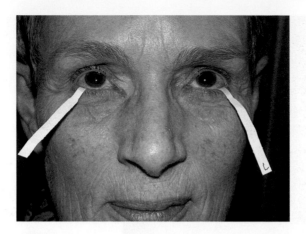

3   Q. Diagnosis of dry eye – true or false?

a. Lack of emotional tearing is uncommon.

b. Frothy tear film.

c. The height of the normal tear meniscus is about 1.5 mm.

d. Tear film break up time of less than 10 seconds is abnormal.

e. Schirmer test (see above) less than 4 mm with anaesthesia is abnormal.

f. There is no clinical test to confirm evaporative KCS.

A.

a. True. **b.** True. **c.** False – about I mm. **d.** True. **e.** False – less than 6 mm with anaesthesia is abnormal. **f.** True.

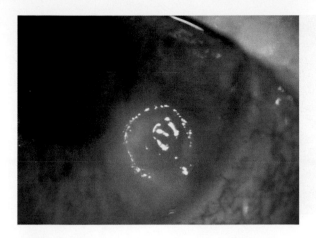

4 Q. Complications of dry eye – true or false?

a. Peripheral superficial corneal neovascularization.

b. Epithelial breakdown.

c. Dellen formation (see above).

d. Viral keratitis.

e. Bacterial keratitis.

f. Perforation.

A.

a. True. **b.** True. **c.** False. **d.** False. **e.** True. **f.** True.

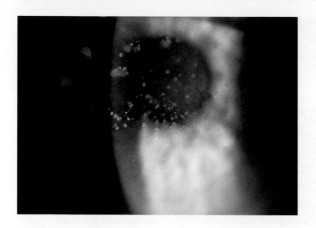

5   **Q. Match the condition (a–f) with the appropriate treatment (i–vi).**

a. Mucin deficiency.

b. Filamentary keratitis (see above).

c. Epithelial defects.

d. Goblet cell deficiency.

e. Posterior blepharitis.

f. Primary Sjögren syndrome.

i. Sodium hyaluronate.

ii. Topical ciclosporin.

iii. Polyvinyl alcohol.

iv. Systemic zidovudine.

v. Systemic tetracycline.

vi. Acetylcysteine 5%.

A.

a. & **iii**; **b.** & **vi**; **c.** & **i**; **d.** & **ii**; **e.** & **v**; **f.** & **iv**.

8

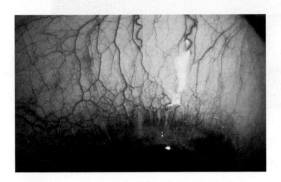

1 Q. Answer the following.

a. What is the lymphatic drainage of the conjunctiva?

b. Where does the palpebral conjunctiva start?

c. What are the palisades of Vogt?

d. Describe the histology of the conjunctival epithelium.

e. Where are goblet cells most dense?

f. At what age does the stroma develop adenoid tissue?

A.

a. To preauricular and submandibular nodes corresponding to the drainage of the eyelids. **b.** At the mucocutaneous junction of the lid margin. **c.** Radial ridges at the limbus (see above). **d.** The epithelium is non-keratinizing and about five cell layers thick. Basal cuboidal cells evolve into flattened polyhedral cells before being shed from the surface **e.** Inferonasally and in the fornices. **f.** About 3 months after birth, hence the inability of the newborn to produce a follicular conjunctival reaction.

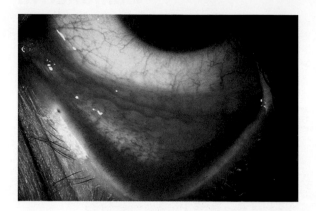

2   Q. The following are associated with follicular conjunctivitis – true or false?

a. Adenoviral conjunctivitis.

b. Parinaud oculoglandular syndrome.

c. Superior limbic keratoconjunctivitis.

d. Adult chlamydial conjunctivitis.

e. Toxic conjunctivitis.

f. Molluscum conjunctivitis.

A.

a. True. **b.** True. **c.** False – papillary. **d.** True. **e.** True. **f.** True.

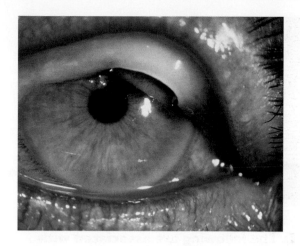

3 **Q. Match the sign (a–f) with the appropriate condition (i–vi).**

a. Mucoid discharge.

b. Serous discharge.

c. Conjunctival haemorrhages.

d. Mucopurulent discharge.

e. Pseudomembranes (see above).

f. Corneal perforation.

i. Acute viral conjunctivitis.

ii. Chlamydial conjunctivitis.

iii. Acute Stevens-Johnson syndrome.

iv. Gonococcal conjunctivitis.

v. Meningococcal conjunctivitis.

vi. Chronic allergic conjunctivitis.

A.

a. & **vi**; b. & **i**; c. & **v**; d. & **ii**; e. & **iii**; f. & **iv**.

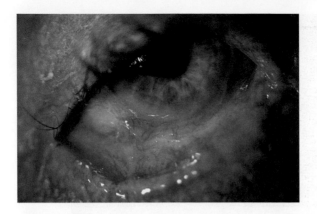

4   **Q. The following are associated with local lymphadenopathy – true or false?**

a. Adenoviral conjunctivitis.

b. Adult chlamydial conjunctivitis.

c. Streptococcal conjunctivitis.

d. Gonococcal conjunctivitis.

e. Parinaud syndrome.

f. Cicatrizing conjunctivitis (see above).

A.

a. True. **b.** True. **c.** False. **d.** True. **e.** True. **f.** False.

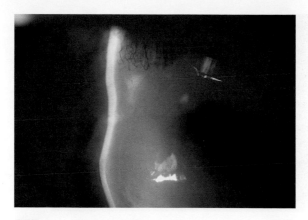

5   Q. Gonococcal keratoconjunctivitis – true or false?

a. *Neisseria gonorrhoeae* can invade the intact corneal epithelium.

b. Laboratory investigations are unnecessary in typical cases.

c. Lymphadenopathy is severe.

d. Corneal involvement usually starts circumferentially.

e. Topical treatment is with gentamicin or bacitracin.

f. Corneal involvement requires oral therapy.

A.

a. True. b. False. c. True. d. False – superiorly (see above). e. True.

f. False – parenteral therapy.

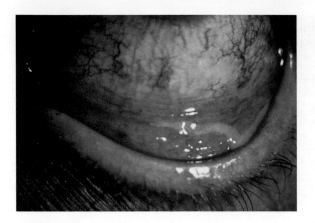

6

Q. Chlamydial conjunctivitis – true or false?

a. It is always bilateral.

b. Discharge is mucopurulent.

c. Conjunctival reaction is follicular.

d. It is associated with non-tender lymphadenopathy

e. Corneal infiltrates may appear within 1 week.

f. Longstanding cases are characterized by more prominent follicles.

A.

a. False – unilateral or bilateral. **b.** True (see above). **c.** True. **d.** False – lymphadenopathy is tender. **e.** False – within 2–3 weeks. **f.** False – less prominent.

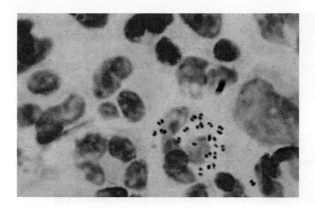

7 Q. Conjunctival smears are not appropriate in the following – true or false?

a. Severe purulent conjunctivitis.

b. Neonatal conjunctivitis.

c. Chronic marginal blepharitis.

d. Follicular conjunctivitis.

e. Papillary conjunctivitis.

f. Bacterial endophthalmitis.

A.

a. False. b. False. c. True. d. False. e. True. f. True.

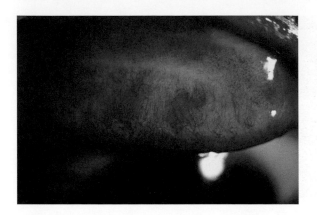

8   Q. Trachoma – answer the following.

a. What is the initial conjunctival reaction in active disease?

b. What are Herbert pits?

c. What is an Arlt line?

d. What is the treatment of active trachoma?

e. What is the SAFE acronym for trachoma control?

f. In the modified WHO grading what does TI signify?

A.

a. Mixed follicular-papillary response. **b.** Shallow depressions at the upper limbus following resolution of follicles. **c.** Scar on the superior tarsal conjunctiva (see above). **d.** Oral azithromycin. **e.** SAFE acronym is Surgery, Antibiotics, Face washing and Environmental improvements. **f.** TI signifies trachomatous inflammation diffusely involving the tarsal conjunctiva, which obscures 50% or more of the normal deep tarsal vessels.

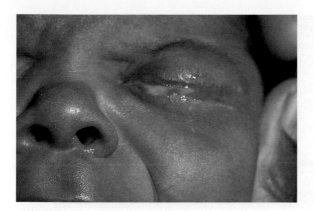

9   Q. Ophthalmia neonatorum – true or false?

a. It is characterized by conjunctivitis within 3 weeks of birth.

b. Conjunctival reaction is follicular.

c. *Chlamydia trachomatis* is the most common causative agent.

d. Chlamydial infection may be associated with pneumonitis.

e. Herpes simplex infection is caused by HSV-2.

f. Topical povidone-iodine 2.5% may be used as prophylaxis.

A.

a. False – 2 weeks. **b.** False – papillary. **c.** True. **d.** True. **e.** True. **f.** True.

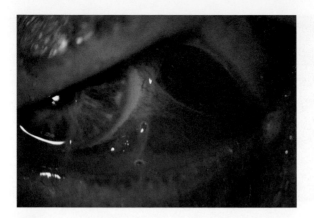

10 **Q. Match the conjunctivitis (a–f) with the appropriate treatment (i–vi).**

a. Chlamydial neonatal conjunctivitis.

b. Gonococcal keratoconjunctivitis.

c. Meningococcal conjunctivitis.

d. Adult chlamydial conjunctivitis.

e. Simple bacterial conjunctivitis.

f. Acute adenoviral conjunctivitis (see above).

i. Parenteral ceftriaxone.

ii. Oral erythromycin.

iii. Oral ciprofloxacin.

vi. Oral doxycycline.

v. Topical fusidic acid.

iv. Symptomatic treatment.

A.

a. & **ii**; **b.** & **i**; **c.** & **iii**; **d.** & **vi**; **e.** & **v**; **f.** & **iv**.

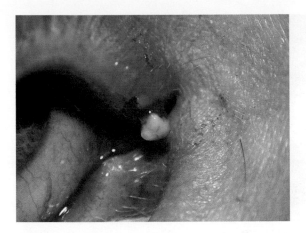

11 Q. Chronic conjunctivitis may be associated with the following – true or false?

a. Floppy eyelid syndrome.

b. Chronic canaliculitis (see above).

c. Chronic dacryoadenitis.

d. Mucus fishing syndrome.

e. Cicatricial pemphigoid.

f. Reiter syndrome.

A.

a. True. **b.** True. **c.** False. **d.** True. **e.** True. **f.** False.

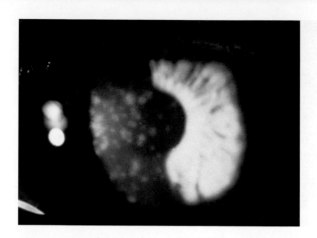

12   Q. Viral keratoconjunctivitis – true or false?

a. Pharyngoconjunctival fever (PCF) is caused by serotypes 3, 8 and 12.

b. Epidemic keratoconjunctivitis (EKC) is caused mainly by serotypes 8, 19 and 37.

c. Keratitis is more common in PCF than EKC.

d. Pseudomembranes may occur.

e. Stage 2 keratitis in EKC is characterized by anterior stromal infiltrates (see above).

f. Molluscum contagiosum conjunctivitis is treated with topical steroids.

A.

a. False – 3, 7 and 11. **b.** True. **c.** False. **d.** True. **e.** False – describes stage 3 keratitis. **f.** False – treated by destroying the eyelid nodule.

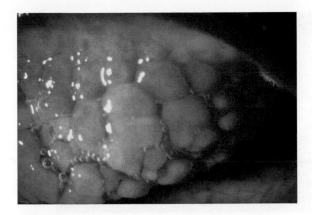

13 Q. Vernal disease – answer the following.

a. In temperate climates, what percentage of patients has associated atopy?

b. How is vernal disease classified?

c. What are giant papillae?

d. What ethnic groups develop limbal vernal disease?

e. What is the usual age at presentation?

f. What are features of decreased disease activity?

A.

a. About 75%. **b.** Classification – palpebral, limbal and mixed. **c.** Giant papillae are larger than 1 mm in diameter and have a flat-topped appearance (see above). **d.** Black and Asian patients. **e.** About 7 years. **f.** Reduction of conjunctival injection and mucus production.

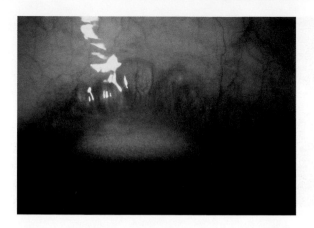

14 **Q. Vernal keratopathy is associated with – true or false?**

a. Superior corneal filaments.

b. Secondary herpes simplex keratitis.

c. Interpalpebral punctate epithelial erosions.

d. Pseudogerontoxon.

e. Shield ulceration.

f. Peripheral neovascularization.

A.

a. False. **b.** True. **c.** False – superior. **d.** True (see above). **e.** True.
f. True.

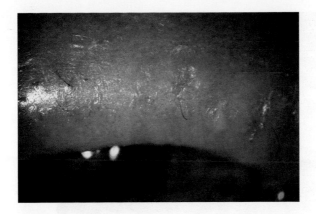

15 **Q. Atopic keratoconjunctivitis is associated with – true or false?**

a. Childhood vernal disease in 5% of cases.

b. Posterior blepharitis.

c. Follicular conjunctivitis involving the inferior fornices.

d. Punctate epithelial keratitis.

e. Forniceal shortening.

f. Predisposition to keratoconus.

A.

a. True. **b.** False – anterior staphylococcal blepharitis and madarosis
(see above). **c.** False – papillary conjunctivitis. **d.** False. **e.** True. **f.** True.

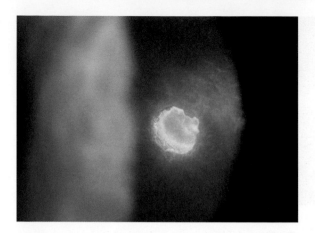

16 Q. Treatment of allergic conjunctivitis – true or false?

a. Lodoxamide is more effective than sodium cromoglicate.

b. Most patients with vernal disease require topical steroids.

c. Systemic ciclosporin may be considered in severe atopic keratoconjunctivitis.

d. Acetylcysteine is useful for early plaque formation (see above) in vernal disease.

e. Supratarsal injection of dexamethasone is as effective as triamcinolone.

f. Giant papillae may require surgical removal.

A.

a. True. b. False. c. True. d. True. e. True. f. False.

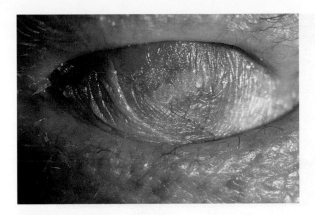

17 Q. Cicatrizing conjunctivitis – answer the following.

a. What is the usual age at presentation of mucous membrane pemphigoid?

b. What two systemic drugs may be used in acute mucous membrane pemphigoid?

c. What is the mean age of onset of Stevens–Johnson disease?

d. What is the pathogenesis of dry eye?

e. What is the pathogenesis of keratopathy (see above)?

f. What is ankyloblepharon?

A.

a. After 70 years of age. **b.** Steroids and cyclophosphamide. **c.** 25 years.

d. Loss of goblet cells and destruction of lacrimal gland orifices.

e. Keratinization, aberrant lashes and infection. **f.** Adhesions at the outer canthus between the upper and lower lids.

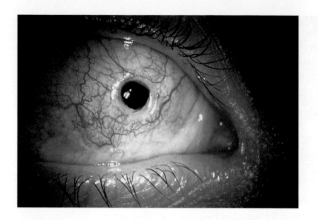

18   Q. Cicatrizing conjunctivitis – true or false?

a. Ocular cicatricial is always bilateral but frequently asymmetrical.

b. Cyclophosphamide should not be used for longer than 12 months because of the risk of liver damage.

c. Patients with acute Stevens–Johnson syndrome must be treated with systemic steroids.

d. Topic retinoic acid is useful for surface drying.

e. End-stage disease is characterized by total symblepharon and corneal opacification.

f. Keratoprostheses are contraindicated in end-stage disease.

A.

a. True. **b.** False – bladder cancer. **c.** False – efficacy of systemic steroids is debatable. **d.** False – to reduce keratinization. **e.** True. **f.** False (see above).

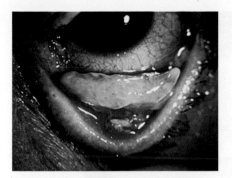

19 Q. Miscellaneous conjunctivitis – true or false?

a. Superior limbic keratoconjunctivitis (SLK) typically affects hyperthyroid females.

b. Most patients with SLK have dry eyes.

c. Ligneous conjunctivitis (see above) presents in childhood.

d. Recurrent ligneous conjunctivitis requires long-term topical acetylcysteine.

e. Parinaud oculoglandular syndrome is characterized by bilateral granulomatous conjunctival lesions.

f. Cat-scratch disease is the most common cause of Parinaud oculoglandular syndrome.

A.

a. True. **b.** False – 50%. **c.** True. **d.** False – ciclosporin and steroids.
e. False – unilateral. **f.** True.

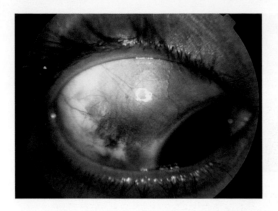

20   Q. Naevus of Ota – true or false?

a. It is usually bilateral.

b. Episcleral pigmentation (see above) can be moved over the sclera.

c. It may be associated with conjunctival melanocytoma.

d. It is an important cause of iris hyperchromia.

e. Iris mamillations are common.

f. The most serious complication is uveal melanoma.

A.

a. False – 5% are bilateral. **b.** False. **c.** False. **d.** True. **e.** False – uncommon. **f.** True.

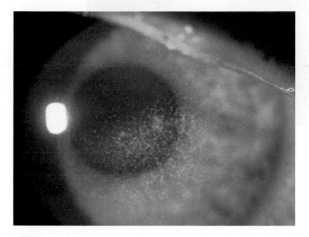

1 **Q. Appropriate location of punctate epithelial erosions – true or false?**

a. Vernal disease – superior.

b. Floppy eyelids – inferior.

c. Lagophthalmos – interpalpebral (see above).

d. Dry eye – interpalpebral.

e. Corneal anaesthesia – superior.

f. Toxicity from drops – inferior.

A.

a. True. **b.** False – superior. **c.** False – inferior. **d.** True. **e.** False – interpalpebral. **f.** True.

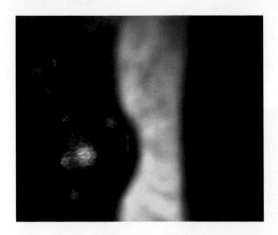

2   **Q. The following are causes of punctate epithelial keratitis – true or false?**

a. Adenoviral infection.

b. Chlamydial infection.

c. Vernal disease.

d. Thygeson disease.

e. Microsporidial keratitis.

f. Acanthamoeba keratitis.

A.

a. True (see above). **b.** True. **c.** False. **d.** True. **e.** True. **f.** False.

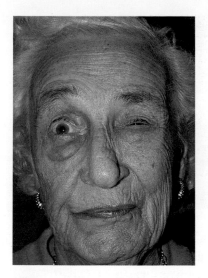

3   Q. The following may cause filamentary keratitis – true or false?

a. Superior limbic keratoconjunctivitis.

b. Sjögren syndrome.

c. Neurotrophic keratitis.

d. Eye patching.

e. Lattice dystrophy.

f. Severe prolonged blepharospasm (see above).

A.

a. True. **b.** True. **c.** True. **d.** True. **e.** False. **f.** True.

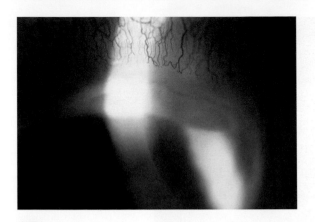

4 Q. Match the description (a–f) with the appropriate condition (i–vi).

a. Small mucus strands lined with epithelium that stains with rose bengal.

b. Tiny epithelial defects that stain with fluorescein.

c. Granular swollen epithelial cells that stain well with rose bengal but poorly with fluorescein.

d. Central stromal and epithelial oedema with underlying keratic precipitates.

e. Superficial neovascularization accompanied by degenerative subepithelial change extending centrally from the limbus.

f. Focal, granular, grey-white opacities usually within the anterior stroma associated with limbal or conjunctival hyperaemia.

i. Punctate epithelial erosions.

ii. Disciform keratitis.

iii. Filamentary keratitis.

iv. Infiltrate (see above).

v. Pannus.

vi. Punctate epithelial keratitis.

A.

a. & **iii**; b. & **i**; c. & **vi**; d. & **ii**; e. & **v**; f. & **iv**.

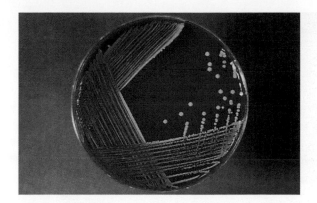

5 **Q. Match the description (a–f) with the appropriate bacterium (i–vi).**

a. Gram-negative kidney-shaped diplococci.

b. Gram-positive cocci arranged in chains.

c. White colonies of coagulase-negative cocci (see above).

d. Golden-yellow colonies of coagulase-positive cocci.

e. Green mucoid colonies of slender Gram-negative rods.

f. Gram-positive club-shaped rods arranged in a Chinese-letter formation.

i. *Staphylococcus epidermidis.*

ii. *Staphylococcus aureus.*

iii. *Neisseria gonorrhoeae.*

iv. *Streptococcus pyogenes.*

v. *Corynebacterium diphtheriae.*

vi. *Pseudomonas aeruginosa.*

A.

a. & **iii**; **b.** & **iv**; **c.** & **i**; **d.** & **ii**; **e.** & **vi**; **f.** & **v**.

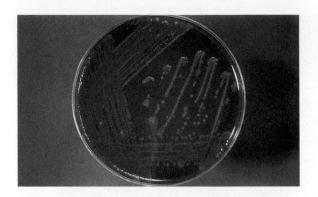

6   **Q. Match each of the micro-organism (a–e) with the appropriate culture medium (i–v).**

a. *Neisseria, Haemophilus* and *Moraxella* spp.

b. *Candida albicans.*

c. *Mycobacterium tuberculosis.*

d. *Acanthamoeba* spp.

e. *Pseudomonas aeruginosa.*

i. *Escherichia coli* plated non-nutrient agar.

ii. Lowenstein–Jensen medium.

iii. Chocolate agar (see above).

iv. Sabouraud dextrose agar.

v. Blood agar.

A.

a. & **iii**; b. & **iv**; c. & **ii**; d. & **i**; e. & **v**.

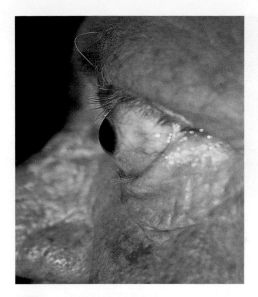

7 Q. The following predispose to bacterial keratitis – true or false?

a. Contact lens wear.

b. Exposure keratopathy.

c. Bullous keratopathy.

d. Neurotrophic keratopathy.

e. Band keratopathy.

f. Atopic keratoconjunctivitis.

A.

a. True. **b.** True (see above). **c.** True. **d.** True. **e.** False. **f.** True.

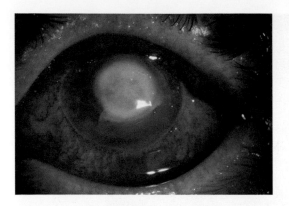

8   Q. Bacterial keratitis – answer the following.

a. Which bacteria are able to penetrate a normal corneal epithelium?

b. What are the most common pathogens?

c. What is the most common risk factor?

d. What is the meaning of intermediate sensitivity to the antimicrobial tested?

e. What are the main characteristics of a bacterial corneal infiltrate?

f. What problem may be associated with topical ciprofloxacin?

A.

a. *Neisseria gonorrhoeae, Neisseria meningitidis, Corynebacterium diphtheriae* and *Haemophilus influenzae*.   **b.** *Pseudomonas aeruginosa, Staphylococcus aureus, Streptococcus pyogenes* and *Streptococcus pneumoniae*.   **c.** Contact lens wear.   **d.** The organism is likely to be sensitive to a high dose of the antimicrobial agent.   **e.** Pain, a central infiltrate more than 1 mm in size associated with an epithelial defect, and anterior uveitis (see above).

f. White corneal precipitates.

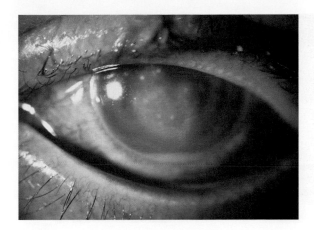

9 Q. Fungal keratitis – answer the following.

a. What are fungi?

b. What are the main types and give examples?

c. Which type is more likely to cause corneal perforation?

d. What is the main risk factor?

e. Are most antifungal agents fungistatic or fungicidal?

f. What is the most commonly used topical antifungal agent?

A.

a. Micro-organisms with rigid walls and multiple chromosomes containing both DNA and RNA. **b.** Filamentous (*Aspergillus* spp., *Fusarium solani*, and *Scedosporium* spp.) and yeasts (*Candida* spp.). **c.** Filamentous fungi. **d.** Trauma with vegetable matter. **e.** Fungistatic. **f.** Econazole 1%.

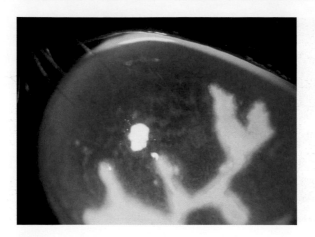

10   Q. Herpes simplex keratitis – true or false?

a. Most cases are caused by HSV-2.

b. Debridement may be used for dendritic ulceration.

c. After the initial episode of epithelial keratitis the risk of recurrence after 1 year is 20%.

d. The virus-laden cells at the margin of a dendritic ulcer stain with fluorescein.

e. Aciclovir is less toxic to the epithelium than vidarabine.

f. Geographic ulceration (see above) may be caused by toxicity to topical antivirals.

A.

a. False – HSV-1. **b.** True. **c.** False – 10%. **d.** False – with rose bengal.
e. True. **f.** False.

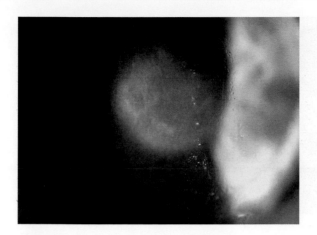

11 Q. Herpes simplex disciform keratitis – true or false?

a. It is caused by a hypersensitivity reaction to viral antigen

b. Past history of dendritic ulceration is the rule.

c. Surrounding Wessely ring develops at the junction of host antigen and viral antibody.

d. Corneal sensation is reduced.

e. Small eccentric lesions do not require treatment.

f. Topical steroids should be avoided.

A.

a. True. **b.** False. **c.** False – viral antigen and host antibody. **d.** True.
e. True. **f.** False.

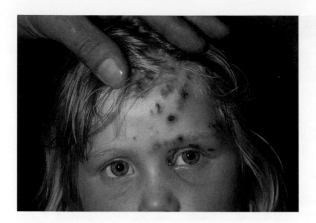

12   Q. Herpes zoster ophthalmicus – true or false?

a. The varicella-zoster virus is antigenically the same but morphologically different from herpes simplex virus.

b. Zoster in a child (see above) may be associated with immunodeficiency or malignancy.

c. Extent of skin rash is related to severity of ocular complications.

d. Initial treatment of acute disease involves oral aciclovir 800 mg five times daily.

e. Nummular keratitis is responsive to topical steroids.

f. Guillain–Barré syndrome may occur during the chronic phase.

A.

a. False – reverse is true. **b.** True. **c.** False. **d.** True. **e.** True. **f.** False – acute phase.

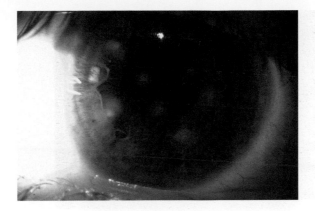

13 **Q. The following occur during the acute stage of herpes zoster ophthalmicus – true or false?**

a. Keratic precipitates.

b. Disciform keratitis.

c. Neurotrophic keratitis

d. Nummular keratitis (see above).

e. Acute epithelial keratitis.

f. Mucous plaque keratitis.

A.

a. True. **b.** True. **c.** False. **d.** True. **e.** True. **f.** False.

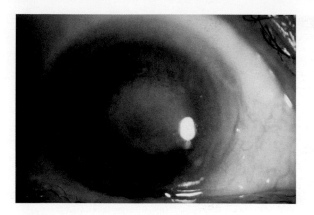

14   Q. Interstitial keratitis (IK) – answer the following.

a. Define IK.

b. What is the most common cause?

c. What is a 'salmon patch'?

d. What is the treatment of active IK?

e. What is the characteristic appearance of healed IK?

f. What is Cogan syndrome?

A.

a. Inflammation of the corneal stroma without primary involvement of the epithelium or endothelium. **b.** Congenital syphilis. **c.** Limbitis associated with deep vascularization of the stroma associated with cellular infiltration and clouding that may obscure the vessels. **d.** Systemic penicillin, topical steroids and cycloplegics. **e.** 'Ghost vessels' with deep stromal scarring and thinning (see above). **f.** Cogan syndrome is characterized by IK and middle ear symptoms.

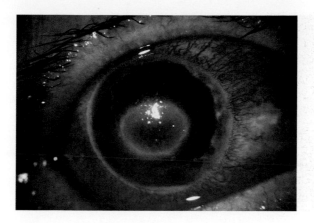

15   Q. Protozoan keratitis – true or false?

a. Acanthamoeba cysts release enzymes that cause cornea destruction.

b. In acanthamoeba keratitis (see above) symptoms are frequently disproportionate to clinical findings.

c. Radial perineuritis is pathognomonic for acanthamoeba keratitis.

d. Initial treatment of acanthamoeba keratitis involves topical Brolene and steroids.

e. Microsporidial keratitis occurs in AIDS.

f. Onchocerciasis may cause sclerosing keratitis.

A.

a. False – trophozoites release enzymes. **b.** True. **c.** True. **d.** False – not steroids. **e.** True. **f.** True.

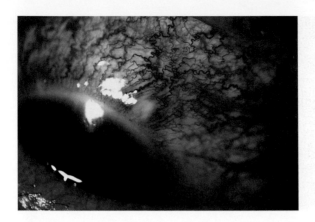

16 Q. Phlyctenular disease – true or false?

a. Is associated with delayed hypersensitivity reaction to bacterial antigens.

b. Typically affects children.

c. Bilateral simultaneous involvement is common.

d. May cause conjunctival scarring.

e. Corneal involvement is rare.

f. Responds readily to topical steroids.

A.

a. True. **b.** True. **c.** False. **d.** False – corneal scarring. **e.** False. **f.** True.

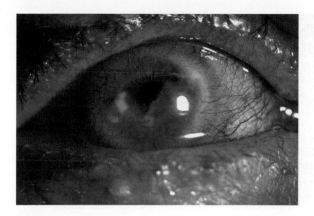

17 Q. Marginal and rosacea keratitis – true or false?

a. Marginal keratitis is often associated with chronic lid margin disease.

b. Marginal keratitis may result in corneal perforation.

c. Recurrent marginal keratitis may require oral tetracycline.

d. Rosacea keratitis (see above) typically occurs in patients with severe facial rosacea.

e. Rosacea keratitis initially involves the superotemporal and superonasal cornea.

f. Rosacea keratitis may result in corneal perforation.

A.

a. True. **b.** False. **c.** True. **d.** False. **e.** False – inferotemporal and inferonasal cornea. **f.** True.

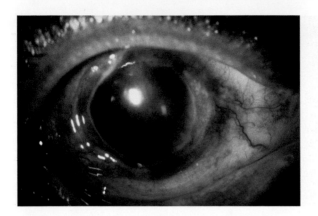

18   Q. Severe peripheral corneal ulceration – answer the following.

a. Define Mooren ulcer.

b. What is the incidence of bilateral involvement in Mooren ulcer?

c. Are there any specific tests for Mooren ulcer?

d. What is the systemic treatment of Mooren ulcer?

e. How does peripheral ulcerative keratitis differ from Mooren ulcer?

f. What are the two most common systemic associations of peripheral ulcerative keratitis?

A.

a. A rare, idiopathic disease characterized by progressive, circumferential, peripheral, stromal ulceration with later central spread (see above).

b. 30%. **c.** No. **d.** Traditionally systemic treatment has been with cyclophosphamide, but more recently ciclosporin has also been shown to be effective. **e.** It may involve the sclera. **f.** Rheumatoid arthritis and Wegener granulomatosis.

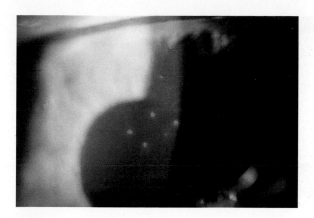

19 Q. Miscellaneous keratitis – true or false?

a. *Streptococcus viridans* is the most common isolate in infectious crystalline keratitis.

b. Infectious crystalline keratitis is usually associated with long-term topical antibiotic therapy.

c. In Thygeson superficial punctate keratitis (see above) the lesions are slightly elevated.

d. Thygeson superficial punctate keratitis is often associated with mild conjunctivitis.

e. Acetylcysteine 2% may be useful in filamentary keratitis.

f. Patching promotes healing and reduces pain in corneal erosions.

A.

a. True. **b.** False – steroid therapy. **c.** True. **d.** False. **e.** False – 5%.
f. False.

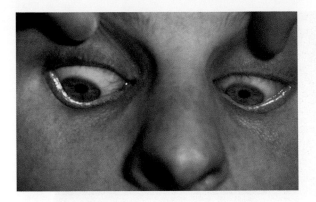

20   **Q. Keratoconus – answer the following questions.**

a. What is keratoconus?

b. How and at what age does it typically present?

c. What is the most sensitive method of detecting early cases?

d. What is Munson sign?

e. What is the pathogenesis of acute hydrops?

f. With which dermatological condition is it associated?

A.

a. A progressive disorder in which the cornea assumes a conical shape secondary to stromal thinning and protrusion. **b.** Typically during puberty with unilateral impairment of vision due to progressive myopia and astigmatism. **c.** Corneal topography. **d.** Bulging of the lower lid in downgaze (see above). **e.** Rupture in Descemet membrane that allows an influx of aqueous into the cornea. **f.** Atopic eczema.

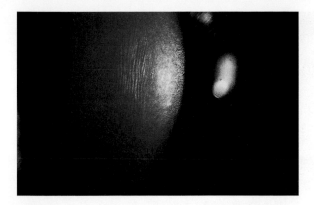

21 Q. The following may occur in keratoconus – true or false?

a. Recurrent corneal erosions.

b. Haab striae.

c. 'Oil droplet' reflex on ophthalmoscopy.

d. Vogt striae.

e. Kayser–Fleischer ring.

f. Reduced corneal sensation.

A.

a. False. **b.** False – occur in congenital glaucoma. **c.** True. **d.** True (see above). **e.** False – occurs in Wilson disease. **f.** False.

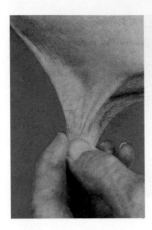

22 **Q. The following systemic conditions are associated with keratoconus – true or false?**

a. Down syndrome.

b. Marfan syndrome.

c. Turner syndrome.

d. Ehlers–Danlos syndrome (see above).

e. Grönblad–Strandberg syndrome.

f. Parry–Romberg syndrome.

A.

a. True. **b.** True. **c.** True. **d.** True. **e.** False. **f.** False.

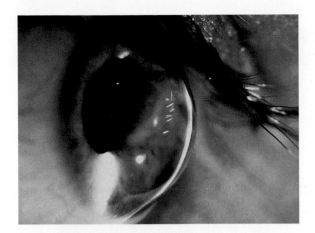

23 Q. Other corneal ectasias – true or false?

a. Pellucid marginal degeneration usually affects the superior cornea.

b. Pellucid marginal degeneration typically presents in early childhood.

c. Pellucid marginal degeneration may be associated with Vogt striae but not acute hydrops.

d. Corneal topography in pellucid marginal degeneration shows a 'butterfly' pattern.

e. Keratoglobus (see above) may be associated with Marfan syndrome.

f. Corneal topography in keratoglobus shows generalized steepening.

A.

a. False – inferior cornea. **b.** False – 4–5th decades. **c.** False. **d.** True.
e. False. **f.** True.

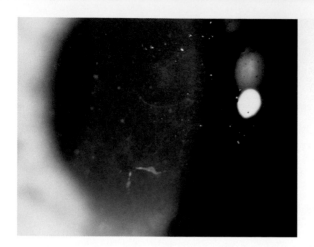

24 Q. Epithelial dystrophies – answer the following.

a. What is the mode of inheritance of epithelial basement membrane dystrophy?

b. What percentage of patients with epithelial basement membrane dystrophy is symptomatic?

c. What are the four types of corneal patterns in epithelial basement membrane dystrophy?

d. What is the mode of inheritance of Meesmann dystrophy?

e. What are the characteristic epithelial changes in Meesmann dystrophy?

f. What is the treatment for Meesmann dystrophy?

A.

a. Usually sporadic and rarely AD. **b.** 10%. **c.** Dots, microcysts, map-like and fingerprint (see above). **d.** AD. **e.** Myriads of tiny intraepithelial cysts of uniform size but variable density maximal centrally and extend towards but do not reach the limbus. **f.** Apart from lubricants treatment is not required.

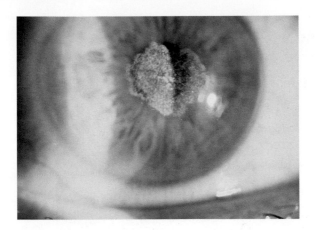

25   Q. Bowman layer dystrophies – true or false?

a. Reis–Bücklers dystrophy typically presents with recurrent corneal erosions.

b. Treatment of Reis–Bücklers dystrophy usually involves lamellar keratoplasty.

c. Thiel–Behnke dystrophy has a honeycomb pattern.

d. Thiel–Behnke dystrophy does not usually require treatment.

e. Schnyder dystrophy (see above) is associated with raised serum cholesterol in 50% of cases.

f. Most cases of Schnyder dystrophy are sporadic.

A.

a. True. **b.** False – excimer laser keratectomy. **c.** True. **d.** True. **e.** True.
f. False – AD.

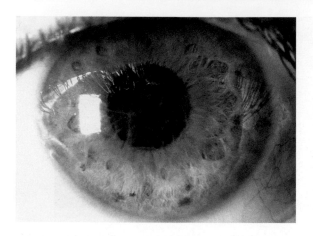

26   Q. Lattice dystrophy – answer the following questions.

a. What is lattice dystrophy?

b. How and when does lattice type 1 present?

c. How does type 2 differ from type 1?

d. What are the systemic features of Meretoja syndrome?

e. Which type is characterized by thick ropy lines extending from limbus to limbus without intervening haze?

f. Which type is initially characterized by anterior stromal, glassy refractile dots?

A.

a. An inherited primary corneal amyloidosis affecting the corneal stroma.

b. End of the first decade with recurrent erosions which precede typical stromal changes. **c.** In type 2 (see above) the lattice lines are more delicate and more radially orientated than in type 1. **d.** Progressive bilateral cranial and peripheral neuropathy, dysarthria, dry, lax itchy skin, characteristic 'mask-like' facial expression due to bilateral facial palsy, and protruding lips and pendulous ears. Amyloidosis may also involve the kidneys and heart.

e. Type 3 and 3A. **f.** Type 1.

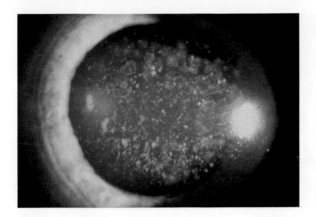

27 Q. Stromal dystrophies – true or false?

a. Inheritance of granular type 1 (see above) is AD with the gene locus on 5q31.

b. Granular dystrophy type 1 presents in the first decade with visual impairment.

c. Granular dystrophy type 2 inevitably requires penetrating keratoplasty.

d. Histology of macular dystrophy shows amorphous hyaline deposits which stain bright red with Masson trichrome.

e. Corneal thinning occurs in advanced macular dystrophy.

f. Corneal grafting should be avoided in gelatinous dystrophy.

A.

a. True. **b.** False – vision is unaffected in the early stages. **c.** False – treatment is not required. **d.** False – refers to macular type 1 dystrophy. **e.** True. **f.** True.

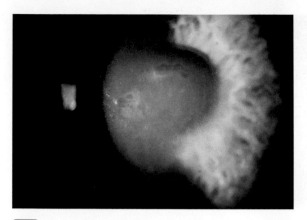

28 Q. Endothelial dystrophies – answer the following.

a. What is Fuchs endothelial dystrophy?

b. What is cornea guttata?

c. What are the characteristics of stage 3 Fuchs dystrophy?

d. What are occasional ocular associations of posterior polymorphous dystrophy?

e. What percentage of eyes with posterior polymorphous dystrophy eventually requires penetrating keratoplasty?

f. What is the underlying defect in congenital hereditary endothelial corneal dystrophy?

A.

a. A bilateral disease characterized by accelerated corneal endothelial cell loss. **b.** Irregular warts or excrescences of Descemet membrane secreted by abnormal endothelial cells. **c.** Bullous keratopathy (see above). **d.** Iris membranes, peripheral anterior synechiae, ectropion uveae, corectopia, polycoria and glaucoma reminiscent of iridocorneal endothelial syndrome. **e.** Nil. **f.** Focal or generalized absence of the corneal endothelium.

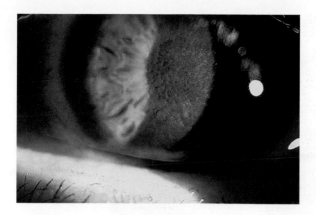

29 Q. The following dystrophies are associated with recurrent corneal erosions – true or false?

a. Meesmann.

b. Epithelial basement membrane.

c. Schnyder.

d. Macular.

e. Thiel–Behnke (see above).

f. Lattice type 1.

A.

a. False. **b.** True. **c.** False. **d.** True. **e.** True. **f.** True.

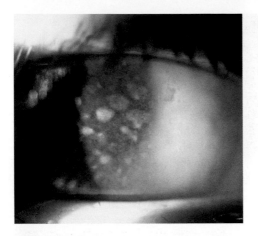

30   **Q. Match the corneal dystrophy (a–f) with appropriate staining or histology (i–vi).**

a. Lattice type 1.

b. Granular type 1.

c. Macular (see above).

d. Reis–Bücklers.

i. Amyloid stained with Congo red.

ii. Glycansaminoglycans stained with Prussian blue and colloidal iron

iii. Amorphous hyaline deposits stained red with Masson trichrome.

iv. Replacement of Bowman layer and epithelial basement membrane with fibrous tissue.

A.

a. & **i**;   **b.** & **iii**;   **c.** & **ii**;   **d.** & **iv**.

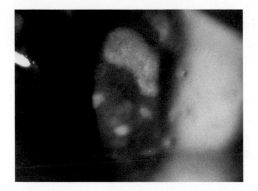

31 Q. Match the description (a–f) with the appropriate corneal degeneration (i–vi).

a. White or yellowish stromal deposits consisting of cholesterol, fats and phospholipids that are not associated with vascularization.

i. Vogt limbal girdle.

b. Amber-coloured granules in the superficial stroma of the peripheral interpalpebral cornea.

ii. Terrien marginal degeneration.

c. Peripheral interpalpebral calcification with clear cornea separating the sharp peripheral margins from the limbus.

iii. Salzmann nodular degeneration.

d. Discrete, elevated grey or blue-grey, nodular, superficial stromal opacities.

iv. Band keratopathy.

e. Fine, yellow-white, punctate stromal opacities frequently associated with mild superficial

v. Spheroidal degeneration.

vascularization, usually start
superiorly, spread circumferentially
and are separated from the limbus
by a clear zone.

f. Bilateral, narrow, crescentic lines
composed of chalk-like flecks
running in the interpalpebral fissure
along the nasal and temporal limbus.

iv. Primary lipid
keratopathy

A.

a. & **vi**; b. & **v**; c. & **iv**; d. & **iii** (see above); e. & **ii**; f. & **i**.

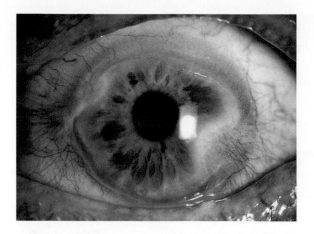

32 Q. Terrien marginal degeneration – true or false?

a. It is usually unilateral.

b. Initially it is asymptomatic and may resemble arcus senilis.

c. Fluorescein staining shows a peripheral epithelial defect.

d. Pterygia may develop in longstanding cases.

e. Poor vision develops in old age due to endothelial decompensation.

f. Penetrating keratoplasty is required to prevent perforation.

A.

a. False – bilateral. **b.** True. **c.** False – epithelium is intact. **d.** False – pseudopterygia (see above). **e.** False – astigmatism. **f.** False.

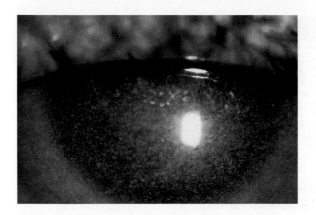

33 **Q. Match the systemic condition (a–f) with the appropriate description of the associated keratopathy (i–vi).**

a. Cystinosis.

i. Numerous, minute, greyish dots throughout the stroma, often concentrated in the periphery in an arcus-like configuration.

b. Wilson disease.

ii. A zone of copper granules in the peripheral part of Descemet membrane.

c. Mucopolysaccharidoses.

iii. Vortex keratopathy.

d. Lecithin-cholesterol-acyltransferase deficiency (Norum disease).

iv. Pseudodendritic lesions.

e. Fabry disease.

v. Corneal crystals.

f. Tyrosinaemia type 2 (Richner–Hanhart syndrome).

vi. Punctate corneal opacification and diffuse stromal haze.

A.

a. & **v** (see above); **b.** & **ii**; **c.** & **vi**; **d.** & **i**; **e.** & **iii**; **f.** & **iv**.

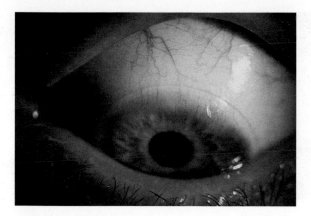

34   Q. Contact lenses complications – answer the following.

a. Which pathogen is most commonly associated with contact lens-related bacterial keratitis?

b. What are the findings in the tight lens syndrome?

c. What are the features of acute contact lens-related red eye?

d. What may be the effects of chronic hypoxia?

e. What are the features of acute toxic keratitis?

f. Which protozoan may cause keratitis in soft contact lens wearers?

A.

a. *Pseudomonas aeruginosa.*   **b.** Indentation and staining of the conjunctival epithelium in a ring around the cornea. **c.** Red eye associated with marginal infiltrates with no or minimal epithelial defects. **d.** Corneal vascularization (see above) and lipid deposition. **e.** Acute pain and redness on lens insertion which may take 48 hours to resolve completely. **f.** *Acanthamoeba* spp.

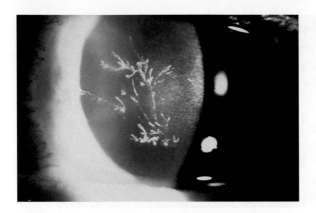

35   **Q. The following are associated with dendritic or pseudodendritic corneal figures – true or false?**

a. Healing corneal abrasion.

b. Herpes zoster ophthalmicus.

c. Adenoviral keratitis.

d. Herpes simplex keratitis.

e. Acanthamoeba keratitis.

f. Cogan dystrophy.

A.

a. True. b. True (see above). c. False. d. True. e. True. f. False.

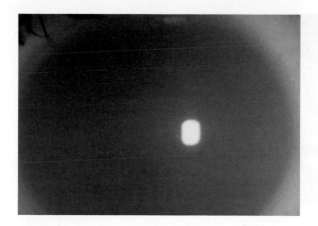

36 **Q. Corneal deposits within the first decade are seen in the following mucopolysaccharidoses – true or false?**

a. Hunter.

b. Sanfilippo.

c. Morquio.

d. Moroteaux Lamy.

e. Hurler.

f. Scheie.

A.

a. False. **b.** False. **c.** False. **d.** True. **e.** True (see above). **f.** True.

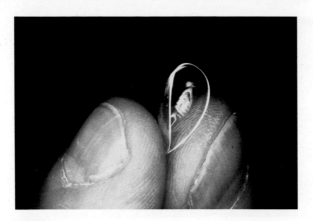

37   **Q. The following are treatment options for recurrent corneal erosions – true or false?**

a. Bandage contact lenses (see above).

b. Debridement.

c. Acetylcysteine.

d. Lubricants.

e. Anterior stromal puncture.

f. Patching.

A.

a. True.   **b.** True.   **c.** False.   **d.** True.   **e.** True.   **f.** False.

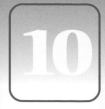

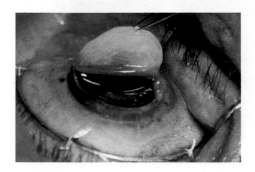

1 Q. Keratoplasty – answer the following.

a. What are the various types of keratoplasty?

b. What is the purpose of tectonic grafting?

c. How soon after death should donor tissue be removed?

d. What is the ideal size of a graft and why?

e. What conditions have the most favourable prognosis for grafting?

f. What is the main advantage of deep lamellar keratoplasty over penetrating?

A.

a. Full-thickness (penetrating – see above) or partial-thickness (lamellar or deep lamellar). **b.** To restore or preserve corneal integrity in eyes with severe structural changes such as stromal thinning and descemetoceles. **c.** Within 24 hours of death. **d.** 7.5 mm; grafts smaller than this may give rise to high astigmatism. **e.** Localized scars, keratoconus and dystrophies. **f.** Decreased risk of rejection because the endothelium is not transplanted.

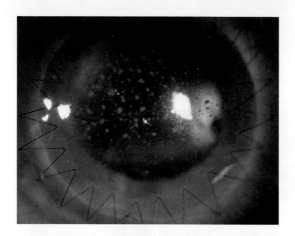

2   Q. Postoperative aspects of keratoplasty – true or false?

a. Sutures are usually removed after 9 months.

b. Topical steroids are often administered once daily for 1 year.

c. Oral aciclovir does not reduce the incidence of recurrence of herpes simplex keratitis.

d. Khodadoust line occurs in endothelial rejection.

e. Subepithelial infiltrates (Krachmer spots) occur in stromal rejection.

f. Urrets–Zavalia syndrome is characterized by persistent miosis.

A.

a. False – 12–18 months. **b.** True. **c.** False. **d.** True. **e.** True (see above).
f. False – mydriasis.

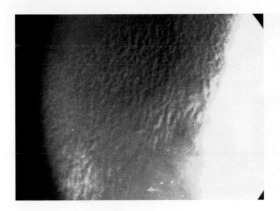

3   Q. Refractive surgery – answer the following.

a. What is refractive surgery?

b. What is the difference between LASIK and LASEK?

c. How much astigmatism can be corrected by photorefractive keratectomy?

d. How much myopia can be corrected by LASIK?

e. What are the main advantages of LASIK over LASEK?

f. What is diffuse lamellar keratitis (sands of Sahara)?

A.

a. A range of procedures aimed at changing the refraction of the eye by altering the cornea and/or crystalline lens, which constitute the principal refracting components. **b.** In LASIK a thin corneal flap is created whereas LASEK the flap involves only epithelium. **c.** Up to 3D of astigmatism. **d.** Up to 12D of myopia, depending on corneal thickness. **e.** LASIK, compared to LASEK, offers the advantages of minimal discomfort, faster visual rehabilitation, rapid stabilization of refraction and minimal stromal haze. **f.** Granular deposits at the flap interface that develop 1–7 days following LASIK (see above).

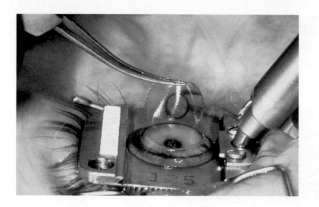

4 Q. Refractive surgery – true or false?

a. LASIK (see above) can correct up to 4D of hypermetropia.

b. In photorefractive keratectomy (PRK) each 10 μm of ablation corrects 1D of myopia.

c. PRK for myopia involves ablation of the peripheral part of the cornea so that it becomes flatter.

d. Laser thermal keratoplasty with a holmium laser can correct low myopia.

e. Conductive keratoplasty with a radiofrequency probe can correct low hypermetropia.

f. During LASIK the central retinal artery may become temporarily occluded and all vision extinguished.

A.

a. True. **b.** True. **c.** False – central cornea. **d.** False - hypermetropia.
e. True. **f.** True.

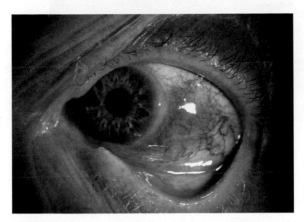

1 **Q. Episcleritis – answer the following.**

a. Within which vascular plexus does maximal congestion occur?

b. How long does a typical attack last?

c. What is the treatment of the first severe attack?

d. What is the treatment of very frequent recurrent attacks?

e. What percentage of patients with recurrent nodular episcleritis (see above) subsequently develops scleritis?

f. What is the purpose of the phenylephrine test?

A.

a. Superficial episcleral plexus. **b.** 3 weeks. **c.** If seen within 48 hours of onset, topical steroids may be used. **d.** Systemic non-steroidal anti-inflammatory drugs. **e.** Nil. **f.** To distinguish nodular episcleritis from nodular scleritis.

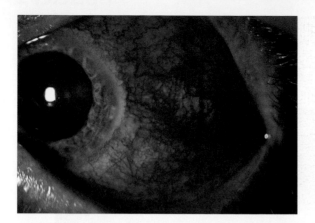

2   Q. Scleritis – answer the following.

a. What is scleritis?

b. What are the main types of anterior non-necrotizing disease?

c. What percentage of patients with non-necrotizing scleritis subsequently develops necrotizing disease?

d. What are specific subtypes of anterior necrotizing disease?

e. What is the usual interval between surgery and the development of surgically-induced scleritis?

f. What is the most common cause of infective scleritis?

A.

a. Oedema and cellular infiltration of the entire thickness of the sclera and may involve adjacent tissues and threaten vision. **b.** Diffuse (see above) and nodular. **c.** 10%. **d.** Vaso-occlusive, granulomatous and surgically-induced. **e.** 3 weeks. **f.** Herpes zoster ophthalmicus.

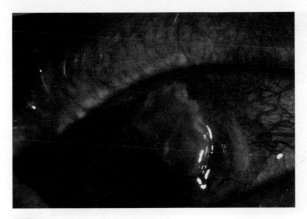

3 **Q. The following are complications of anterior necrotizing scleritis with inflammation – true or false?**

a. Glaucoma.

b. Bacterial endophthalmitis.

c. Peripheral ulcerative keratitis.

d. Hypotony.

e. Secondary fungal infection.

f. Uveitis.

A.

a. True. **b.** False. **c.** True (see above). **d.** True. **e.** False. **f.** True.

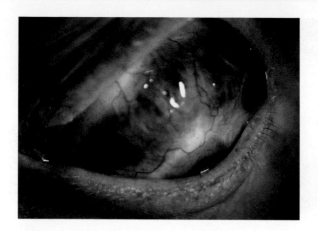

4   Q. Scleromalacia perforans – true or false?

a. It typically affects men with Wegener granulomatosis.

b. It may be detected by chance.

c. It is nearly always preceded by necrotizing scleritis with inflammation.

d. Spontaneous scleral perforation eventually occurs in 15% of longstanding cases.

e. Treatment involves systemic steroids.

f. Scleral grafts should be performed without delay in unresponsive cases.

A.

a. False – women with sero-positive rheumatoid arthritis. **b.** True.
c. False. **d.** False. **e.** False. **f.** False.

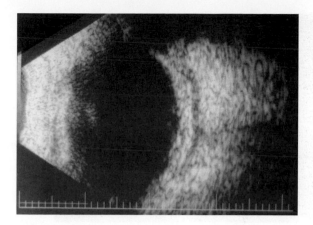

5   Q. Posterior scleritis – true or false?

a. Young patients are usually healthy.

b. About 25% of eyes develop exudative retinal detachment.

c. Fluorescein angiography is of more diagnostic value than ultrasonography.

d. It may cause proptosis.

e. Associated anterior scleritis is uncommon.

f. Prognosis is not as good as in anterior scleritis.

A.

a. True. **b.** True. **c.** False – reverse applies (see above). **d.** True. **e.** False.
f. True.

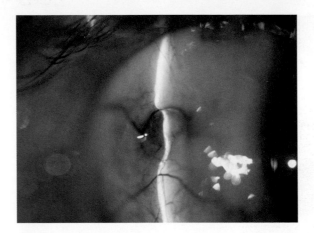

6   **Q. Treatment of scleritis – true or false?**

a. Most patients do not require treatment.

b. Periocular steroids should never be used.

c. Topical steroids may relieve symptoms and oedema in non-necrotizing disease.

d. Systemic non-steroidal anti-inflammatory agents should be used only in non-necrotizing disease.

e. All patients with necrotizing disease (see above) require systemic cytotoxic agents.

f. Systemic ciclosporin may be useful as short-term therapy.

A.

a. False. **b.** False – may be used in non-necrotizing anterior disease.
c. True. **d.** True. **e.** False – only if systemic steroids fail or as steroid-sparing agents. **f.** True.

12

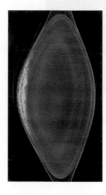

1 Q. Acquired cataract – answer the following.

a. Which type of age-related cataract frequently affects reading vision more than distance?

b. Which type of age-related cataract may give rise to 'second sight of the aged'?

c. Which type of age-related cataract typically gives rise to glare due to light scattering?

d. What is a mature cataract?

e. What is a hypermature cataract?

f. What is a morgagnian cataract?

A.

a. Posterior subcapsular (see above). **b.** Nuclear. **c.** Cortical. **d.** A completely opaque lens. **e.** A cataract with a shrunken and wrinkled anterior capsule due to leakage of water out of the lens. **f.** A hypermature cataract in which liquefaction of the cortex has allowed the nucleus to sink inferiorly.

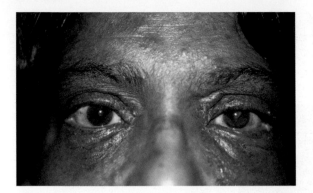

2   **Q. Systemic associations of acquired cataract – true or false?**

a. Classical diabetic cataract is characterized by snowflake nuclear opacities.

b. About 90% of patients with myotonic dystrophy develop cataract in the third decade of life.

c. Occasionally cataract may antedate myotonia.

d. About 10% of patients with severe atopic dermatitis (see above) develop cataract in the second to third decades.

e. Cataracts in atopic dermatitis are usually mild and non-progressive.

f. Neurofibromatosis-1 is associated with presenile cataract.

A.

a. False – snowflake cortical opacities. **b.** True. **c.** True. **d.** True. **e.** False.
f. False – neurofibromatosis-2.

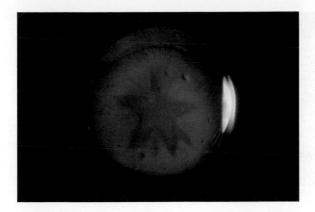

3 Q. Match the cataract (a–f) with the appropriate condition (i–vi).

a. Shield-like anterior subcapsular.

b. Snowflake.

c. Stellate posterior subcapsular (see above).

d. Sun-flower.

e. Spoke-like posterior.

f. Oil droplet.

i. Mannosidosis.

ii. Diabetes.

iii. Atopic dermatitis.

iv. Myotonic dystrophy.

v. Wilson disease.

vi. Galactosaemia.

A.

a. & iii; b. & ii; c. & i; d. & v; e. & i; f. & vi.

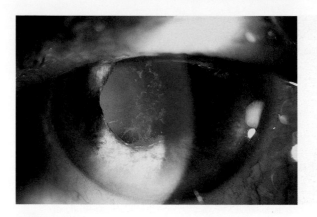

4   **Q. Secondary (complicated) cataract – true or false?**

a. Secondary cataract develops as a result of some other primary ocular disease.

b. Chronic anterior uveitis is the most common cause of secondary cataract.

c. Fuchs uveitis syndrome may present with bilateral secondary cataract.

d. Polychromatic lustre at the anterior pole of the lens is often the earliest finding in secondary cataract.

e. Glaukomflecken is pathognomonic for a previous attack of acute angle-closure glaucoma.

f. Cataract surgery is unlikely to improve vision in patients with retinitis pigmentosa.

A.

a. True. **b.** True. **c.** False – unilateral. **d.** False – posterior pole. **e.** True (see above). **f.** False.

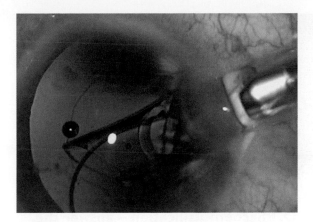

5   Q. Cataract surgery – answer the following.

a. What is the most common indication for cataract surgery?

b. Approximately how many dioptres are subtracted from the refracting system of the eye by cataract surgery?

c. Which two parameters are measured in biometry?

d. What are the two currently used biometric methods?

e. What is the size of the incision required to insert a rigid intraocular lens (IOL)?

f. What are the main types of flexible IOLs (see above)?

A.

a. Visual improvement. **b.** 20D **c.** Keratometry and measurement of the axial length. **d.** A-scan ultrasonic biometry and Zeiss IOL Master. **e.** More than 5 mm. **f.** Silicone, acrylic and hydrogel.

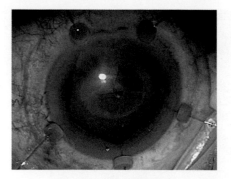

6   Q. Phacoemulsification – answer the following.

a. What is the concentration of povidone-iodine?

b. What two vectors are involved in capsulorrhexis?

c. How may visualization of the anterior capsule be enhanced in a mature cataract?

d. What is the purpose of hydrodissection?

e. What may occur from too vigorous hydrodissection?

f. What is the meaning of 'divide and conquer'?

A.

a. 5%. **b.** Tangential vector (shearing) and a centripetal vector (ripping).

c. The anterior capsule can be stained with trypan blue (see above).

d. So that the nucleus can be more easily and safely rotated thus reducing zonular stress. **e.** Rupture of the posterior capsule. **f.** The nucleus is separated into four quadrants and then each quadrant is emulsified and aspirated.

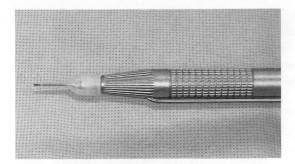

7   Q. Phacoemulsification – true or false?

a. Aspiration flow rate refers to the volume of fluid removed from the eye in ml/minute.

b. The Venturi pump pulls liquid and lens material into the phaco tip by milking fluid filled tubing over rollers.

c. The phaco handpiece (see above) contains a series of piezo electric crystals which act as rapid switching devices to enable the tip to vibrate longitudinally at ultrasonic frequencies.

d. The jackhammer pneumatic drill effect does not significantly contribute to breaking up lens material.

e. Viscoelastics are tripolymers whose main constituents are glycansaminoglycans and hydroxypropylmethylcellulose.

f. Dispersive viscoelastics have long chains and a high molecular weight.

A.

a. True. **b.** False – refers to a peristaltic pump. **c.** True. d. False. **e.** False – bipolymers. **f.** False – cohesive viscoelastics.

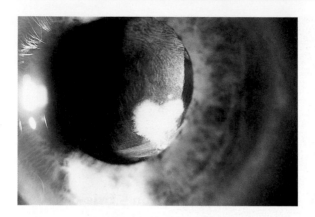

8   Q. Postoperative endophthalmitis – answer the following.

a. What percentage of acute bacterial endophthalmitis is caused by Gram-negative organisms?

b. What culture media should be used?

c. What are the antibiotics and their concentrations that can be injected intravitreally in acute bacterial endophthalmitis?

d. What is the main criterion for pars plana vitrectomy in acute bacterial endophthalmitis?

e. What pathogens may cause delayed-onset endophthalmitis?

f. What is the characteristic appearance of the posterior capsule in delayed-onset endophthalmitis?

A.

a. About 10% are caused by Gram-negative organisms. **b.** Blood agar, cooked meat broth and brain–heart infusion. **c.** Ceftazidime (2 mg in 0.1 ml), vancomycin (2 mg in 0.1 ml) and amikacin (0.5 mg in 0.1 ml). **d.** Visual acuity of light perception. **e.** The most common is *Propionibacterium acnes* and occasionally *Staphylococcus epidermidis*, *Corynebacterium* spp. or *Candida parapsilosis*. **f.** Enlarging white capsular plaque (see above).

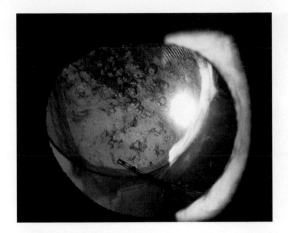

9   Q. Postoperative capsular opacification – true or false?

a. It is the most common late complication of cataract surgery.

b. Capsular fibrosis is more common than Elschnig pearls (see above).

c. Laser capsulotomy may precipitate chronic endophthalmitis.

d. Initial setting in laser capsulotomy is 1 mJ/pulse.

e. Glaucoma is the most serious complication of laser capsulotomy.

f. Capsulotomy opening of about 5 mm is usually adequate.

A.

a. True. **b.** False – reverse applies. **c.** True. **d.** True. **e.** False – retinal detachment. **f.** False – about 3 mm.

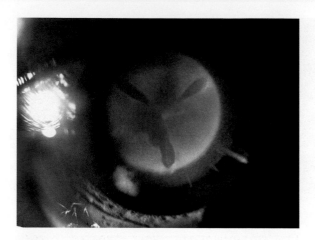

10   Q. Congenital cataract – answer the following.

a. What percentage of cases is bilateral?

b. What is the most common mode of inheritance?

c. What is the systemic condition most frequently associated with co-existent congenital cataract and congenital glaucoma?

d. What are 'riders'?

e. Which intrauterine infections may be associated with cataract?

f. What is the most common chromosomal abnormality associated with cataract?

A.

a. About 66%. **b.** AD. **c.** Lowe syndrome – 100% cataract; 50% glaucoma. **d.** Radial extensions from a lamellar cataract (see above).

e. Rubella, cytomegalovirus, herpes simplex, toxoplasmosis and varicella.

f. Trisomy 21 (Down syndrome).

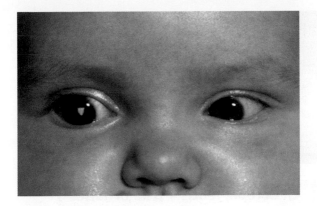

11 Q. Congenital cataract – true or false?

a. In galactosaemia the exclusion of galactose (in milk products) from the diet does not prevent the progression of cataract.

b. The rubella virus is capable of persisting in the lens for up to 3 years after birth.

c. Bilateral dense cataracts require at surgery 4–6 weeks of age.

d. Surgery for dense unilateral cataracts (see above) is performed mainly for cosmetic reasons.

e. Postoperative posterior capsular opacification is rare in children.

f. Intraocular lenses should never be used in infants.

A.

a. False. **b.** True. **c.** True. **d.** False – should be performed urgently.
e. False. **f.** False.

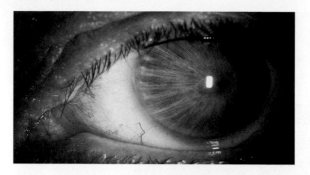

12   Q. Ectopia lentis – true or false?

a. Ectopia lentis refers to a complete dislocation of the lens from its normal position.

b. Familial ectopia lentis is characterized by bilateral symmetrical superotemporal displacement.

c. In ectopia lentis et pupillae (see above) the lens and pupil are displaced in the same direction.

d. All patients with Marfan syndrome eventually develop ectopia lentis.

e. Most patients with homocystinuria and ectopia lentis maintain accommodation.

f. In homocystinuria the dislocation is usually inferiorly.

A.

a. False – may be partial. **b.** True. **c.** False – in opposite directions.
d. False – about 80%. **e.** False – zonules becomes disintegrated and accommodation lost. **f.** True.

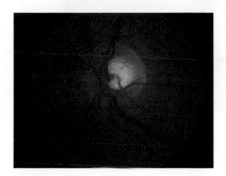

1   Q. Normal optic nerve head – answer the following.

a. Which part of the neuroretinal rim is the broadest?

b. What is the rim–disc ratio?

c. What is the cup–disc ratio?

d. What is the vertical cup–disc in the majority of normal eyes?

e. What is the zone beta?

f. What is the zone alpha?

A.

a. Inferior – remember ISNT (inferior, superior, nasal and temporal – see above). **b.** Thickness of the rim in four quadrants expressed as a fraction of the diameter of the disc. **c.** Diameter of the cup expressed as a fraction of the diameter of the disc which should be measured in both vertical and horizontal meridia. **d.** 0.3 or less. **e.** Area of chorioretinal atrophy that borders the disc margin. **f.** It concentrically surrounds zone beta and is characterized by hyper- and hypopigmentation of the retinal pigment epithelium.

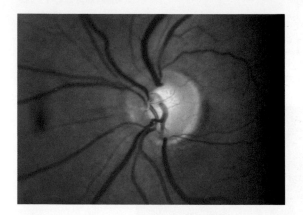

2   **Q. Glaucomatous optic neuropathy – true or false?**

a. Zone alpha is larger and occurs more frequently in patients with primary open-angle glaucoma (POAG).

b. Focal ischaemic (type 1) discs are characterized by polar notching that may be associated with localized field defects near fixation.

c. Myopic glaucomatous (type 2) discs typically affect elderly females with low-tension glaucoma.

d. Senile sclerotic (type 3) discs tend to occur in patients with ischaemic heart disease and hypertension.

e. Bayoneting is characterized by a space between a superficial blood vessel that runs from the superior or inferior aspects of the disc towards the macula, and the disc margin.

f. Disc haemorrhages may antedate visual field defects.

A.

a. False – refers to zone beta. **b.** True (see above). **c.** False – young patients, particularly males. **d.** True. **e.** False – refers to baring of circumlinear blood vessels. **f.** True.

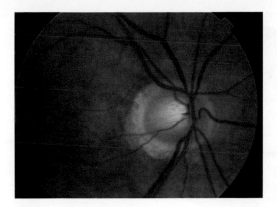

3   Q. Ocular hypertension – true or false?

a. 15% of individuals over the age of 40 years have an intraocular pressure (IOP) greater than 21 mmHg.

b. Over 30% of ganglion cells have to be lost before damage can be detected by conventional perimetry.

c. Parapapillary changes (see above) are present in 50% of ocular hypertensives who subsequently convert to POAG.

d. In patients with ocular hypertension, a family history of POAG in a first degree relative is a high risk factor for subsequent conversion to POAG.

e. Cumulative risk of an untreated ocular hypertensive developing POAG after 5 years is 20%.

f. Vertical cup–disc ratio of 0.4 or more and central corneal thickness of 555–588 μm is a high risk factor for POAG.

A.

a. False – 7%. **b.** False – 20%. **c.** True. **d.** False – moderate risk factor.
e. False – 9.5%. **f.** False – moderate risk factor.

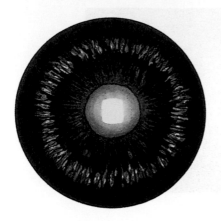

 Q. Steroid responsiveness – true or false?

a. Steroid non-responders account for about 40% of the general population.

b. About 75% of patients with POAG are high responders.

c. Topical prednisolone has a lesser propensity for raising intraocular pressure than dexamethasone.

d. Fluorometholone raises intraocular pressure half as much as betamethasone.

e. Systemic steroids raise intraocular pressure as much as topical steroids.

f. Patients with pigment dispersion syndrome (see above) have an increased incidence of steroid responsiveness.

A.

a. False – 60%. **b.** False – 90%. **c.** False – equal. **d.** True. **e.** False – less. **f.** True.

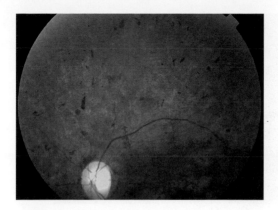

5   Q. POAG – answer the following.

a. What is POAG?

b. What is the prevalence of POAG in the general population over the age of 40 years?

c. What percentage of patients with POAG has IOP below 22 mmHg?

d. Who carries a greater risk, offspring or siblings of patients with POAG?

e. What two genes have so far been identified for POAG?

f. What other ocular diseases are associated with an increased risk of POAG?

A.

a. A neurodegenerative disease of the optic nerve characterized by accelerated ganglion cell death, subsequent axonal loss and optic nerve damage, and eventual visual field loss. **b.** About 1%. **c.** About 16%. **d.** Siblings have a 10% and offspring a 4% risk. **e.** The myocilin gene (MYOC) on chromosome 1q21-q31 and the optineurin gene in the GLC-1E interval on chromosome 10p. **f.** Myopia, Fuchs endothelial dystrophy, retinitis pigmentosa (see above), central retinal vein occlusion and rhegmatogenous retinal detachment.

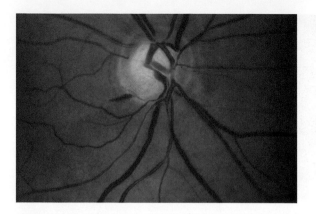

6   Q. Normal tension glaucoma – true or false?

a. It is nearly as common as POAG.

b. Patients are significantly older than those with POAG.

c. IOP is usually in the lower teens.

d. Splinter-shaped disc haemorrhages (see above) are more common than in POAG.

e. Without treatment progression of visual field loss is inevitable.

f. Trabeculectomy is the only effective form of treatment.

A.

a. False – much less common. **b.** True. **c.** False – usually in the upper teens. **d.** True. **e.** False – without treatment 40% of patients show no progression after 5 years. **f.** False – many can be controlled medically.

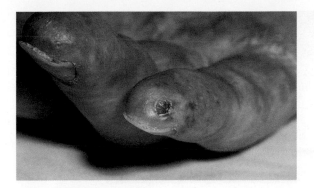

7 Q. Characteristics of patients with normal tension glaucoma – true or false?

a. Male.

b. Systemic hypertension.

c. Raynaud phenomenon (see above).

d. Migraine.

e. Paraproteinaemia and serum autoantibodies

f. Japanese.

A.

a. False. **b.** False. **c.** True. **d.** True. **e.** True. **f.** True.

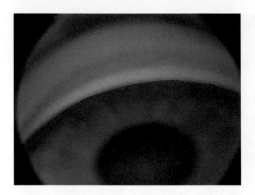

8   Q. Primary angle-closure glaucoma (PACG) – answer the following.

a. What is primary angle closure?

b. What is PACG?

c. What is the female:male ratio?

d. What is the average age at presentation?

e. Why are first degree relatives at increased risk?

f. What does gonioscopy show in an angle closure suspect?

A.

a. This occurs in anatomically predisposed eyes, without other pathology, in which vision is threatened by elevation of IOP, as a consequence of obstruction of aqueous outflow by occlusion of the trabecular meshwork by the peripheral iris. **b.** PACG is a term that should be used only when primary angle closure has resulted in optic nerve damage and visual field loss. **c.** 4:1. **d.** 60 years. **e.** Because predisposing anatomical factors are frequently inherited. **f.** 'Occludable' angle in which the pigmented trabecular meshwork is not visible in at least three quadrants (Shaffer grade 1 or 0 – see above).

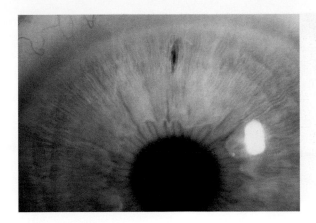

9 Q. PACG – true or false?

a. It is the most common type of glaucoma in black patients.

b. Eyes with PACG have a corneal diameter 0.25 mm smaller than normal.

c. In patients with haloes associated with intermittent angle closure, the blue end of the spectrum is nearer to the source of light.

d. All patients with intermittent angle closure must have laser iridotomy (see above).

e. Immediate treatment of acute angle closure involves instillation of pilocarpine 2%.

f. Laser iridotomy is effective in lowering IOP in 75% of cases of acute angle closure.

A.

a. False – Chinese. **b.** True. **c.** True. **d.** True. **e.** False. **f.** True.

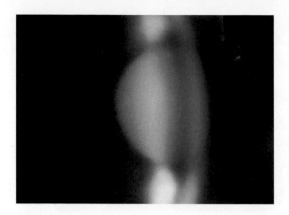

10 **Q. These conditions need to be considered in differential diagnosis of acute congestive PACG – true or false?**

a. Neovascular glaucoma.

b. Angle-recession glaucoma.

c. Phacomorphic glaucoma.

d. Migrainous neuralgia.

e. Posner–Schlossman syndrome

f. Plateau iris syndrome.

A.

a. True. **b.** False – glaucoma is chronic. **c.** True (see above). **d.** True.
e. True. **f.** True.

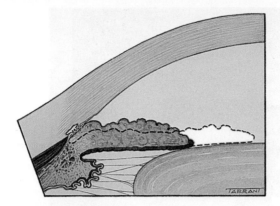

11 Q. Plateau iris syndrome – true or false?

a. The iris plane is flat and the central anterior chamber depth normal.

b. Inheritance is AD.

c. It is characterized by acute angle-closure glaucoma without pupillary block.

d. It occurs in the same age group as angle closure with pupillary block.

e. Angle closure develops despite a patent iridotomy.

f. Laser trabeculoplasty is effective in early cases.

A.

a. True (see above). **b.** False. **c.** True. **d.** False – younger. **e.** True.
f. False.

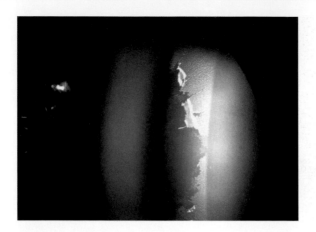

12 Q. Pseudoexfoliation – answer the following.

a. Which European race is at particular risk?

b. What is the composition of pseudoexfoliative material (see above)?

c. What is Sampaolesi line?

d. Why is cataract surgery more hazardous?

e. Why is the visual prognosis less good than in POAG?

f. What is the cumulative risk of glaucoma in an eye with pseudoexfoliation at 5 and 10 years?

A.

a. Scandinavians. **b.** Grey-white, fibrillogranular, extracellular matrix composed of a protein core surrounded by glycosaminoglycans.

c. Scalloped band of pigment running on to or anterior to Schwalbe line.

d. Because of poor mydriasis, and an increased risk of vitreous loss due to zonulodialysis. **e.** Because the IOP is often significantly elevated and may also exhibit great fluctuation so that severe damage may develop rapidly.

f. 5% at 5 years; 15% at 10 years.

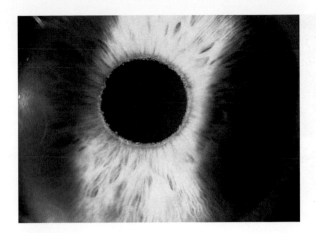

13 Q. Pseudoexfoliation – true or false?

a. Pseudoexfoliative material on the pupillary border is common.
b. Trabecular hyperpigmentation is most marked superiorly.
c. Occasionally the IOP may rise acutely despite the angle being wide open.
d. Laser trabeculoplasty is less effective than in POAG.
e. Trabeculectomy has the same success rate as in POAG.
f. Presentation is earlier than POAG.

A.

a. True (see above). **b.** False – inferiorly. **c.** True. **d.** False. **e.** True.
f. False.

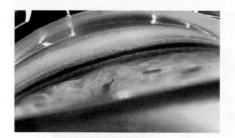

14   Q. Pigment dispersion syndrome – answer the following.

a. What is pigment dispersion syndrome?

b. What is the cause of pigment shedding?

c. What are the characteristics of patients most at risk?

d. How does trabecular hyperpigmentation differ from that in pseudoexfoliation?

e. What is the pathogenesis of elevation of IOP?

f. What is the incidence of elevation of IOP after 15 years?

A.

a. It is characterized by the liberation of pigment granules from the iris pigment epithelium and their deposition throughout the anterior segment.
b. Mechanical rubbing of the posterior pigment layer of the iris against packets of lens zonules as a result of excessive posterior bowing of the mid-peripheral portion of the iris.   **c.** Young myopic men.   **d.** Pigment is finer than in pseudoexfoliation and appears to lie both on and within the trabecular meshwork. It also has a more homogeneous appearance and forms a dense band involving the entire circumference of the meshwork uniformly (see above).   **e.** Pigmentary obstruction of the intertrabecular spaces and damage to the trabeculum secondary to denudation, collapse and sclerosis.   **f.** About 30%.

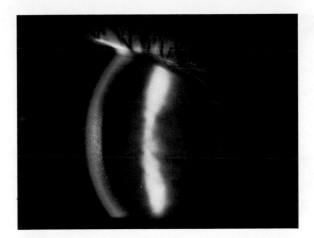

15 Q. Pigment dispersion syndrome – true or false?

a. Most patients are hypermetropic and have shallow anterior chambers.

b. The condition is more common in blacks than whites.

c. Strenuous exercise may result in elevation of IOP.

d. Krukenberg spindle (see above) is neither universal nor pathognomonic.

e. Gonioscopy shows a wide open angle with characteristic midperipheral iris concavity that may increase with accommodation.

f. Initial IOP, cup–disc ratio and degree of trabecular hyperpigmentation are helpful in identifying those who will eventually develop glaucoma.

A.

a. False – are myopic and have deeper than normal anterior chambers.

b. False – rare in blacks. **c.** True. **d.** True. **e.** True. **f.** False.

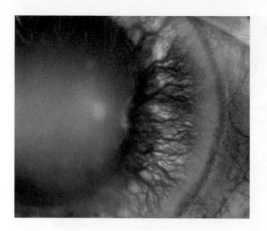

16   **Q. The following conditions are associated with rubeosis iridis – true or false?**

a. Chronic anterior uveitis.

b. Carotid obstructive disease.

c. Longstanding retinal detachment.

d. Iris naevus syndrome.

e. Choroidal melanoma.

f. Sturge–Weber syndrome.

A.

a. True. **b.** True. **c.** True. **d.** False. **e.** True. **f.** False.

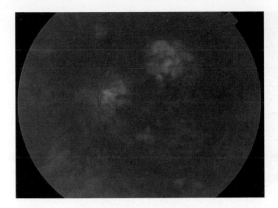

17 Q. Neovascular glaucoma – true or false?

a. Diabetes is the most common cause of rubeosis iridis.

b. Glaucoma typically develops 6 months after an ischaemic central retinal vein occlusion (see above).

c. Angle neovascularization may occur without pupillary involvement by new vessels.

d. Central retinal artery occlusion is never associated with rubeosis iridis.

e. The main aim of treatment of severe neovascular glaucoma is to relieve pain, as the prognosis for maintaining visual function is extremely poor.

f. Trans-scleral diode laser cycloablation should never be performed in advanced neovascular glaucoma.

A.

a. False – ischaemic central retinal vein occlusion. **b.** False – 3 months.
c. True. **d.** False. **e.** True. **f.** False.

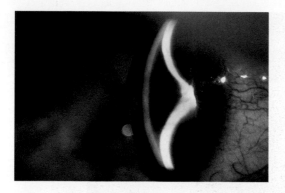

18   Q. Inflammatory glaucoma – true or false?

a. A common cause of raised IOP in individuals with ocular inflammation is the use of systemic steroids.

b. Ciliary body shutdown caused by acute exacerbation of chronic anterior uveitis is frequently associated with lowering of IOP that may mask the underlying tendency to glaucoma.

c. Most eyes with seclusio pupillae (see above) exhibit a normal or subnormal IOP due to concomitant chronic ciliary body shutdown.

d. In acute anterior uveitis the IOP is usually moderately elevated.

e. In angle-closure glaucoma without pupil block, the anterior chamber is shallow and gonioscopy shows extensive angle closure by PAS.

f. Posner–Schlossman syndrome (glaucomatocyclitic crisis) is characterized by recurrent attacks of bilateral, acute secondary open-angle closure glaucoma associated with mild anterior uveitis.

A.

a. False – topical steroids. **b.** True. **c.** True. **d.** False – IOP is usually normal or subnormal due to concomitant ciliary shutdown. **e.** False – applies to angle-closure glaucoma with pupil block. **f.** False – unilateral and the glaucoma is of the open-angle type.

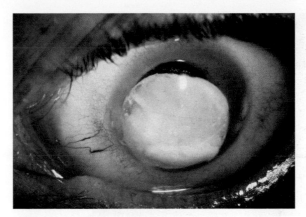

19 Q. Lens-related glaucoma – true or false?

a. Phacolytic glaucoma (lens protein glaucoma) is a closed-angle glaucoma occurring in association with a hypermature cataract.

b. In phacolytic glaucoma trabecular obstruction is caused by high molecular weight lens proteins which have leaked through the intact capsule into the aqueous humour.

c. Phacomorphic glaucoma is an acute secondary angle-closure glaucoma precipitated by an intumescent cataractous lens.

d. Initial treatment of phacomorphic glaucoma involves cataract surgery.

e. Trivial ocular trauma in homocystinuria may result in lens dislocation into the anterior chamber.

f. Treatment of acute pupil block by a hard lens dislocated into the anterior chamber (see above) involves intracapsular cataract extraction.

A.

a. False – open-angle glaucoma. **b.** True. **c.** True. **d.** False – initial treatment is similar to acute PACG. **e.** True. **f.** True.

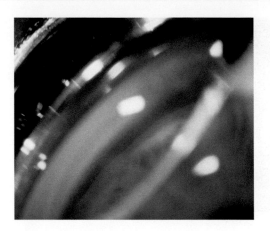

20 Q. Traumatic glaucoma – true or false?

a. Hyphaema in a diabetic patient is more likely to give rise to elevation of IOP.

b. In red cell glaucoma the optic nerve is endangered by IOP >50 mmHg for 2 days.

c. Topical steroids should never be used in red cell glaucoma.

d. Less than 10% of eyes with angle recession develop glaucoma after 10 years.

e. The risk of glaucoma is not related to the extent of angle recession (see above).

f. Trabeculectomy with adjunctive antimetabolites is the most effective treatment for severe angle-recession glaucoma.

A.
a. False. **b.** True. **c.** False. **d.** True. **e.** False. **f.** True.

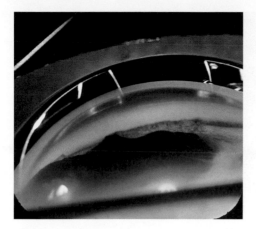

21   Q. Iridocorneal endothelial (ICE) syndrome – true or false?

a. It is bilateral but involvement is often asymmetrical.

b. Middle-aged women are typically affected.

c. Glaucoma is caused by synechial angle closure secondary to contraction of abnormal corneal endothelium tissue.

d. Chandler syndrome may present with corneal oedema.

e. Cogan–Reese syndrome may be associated with iris melanoma.

f. Artificial filtering shunts are eventually required in many cases with glaucoma.

A.

a. False – always unilateral. **b.** True. **c.** True (see above). **d.** True.

e. False – associated with diffuse iris naevus or iris nodules. **f.** True.

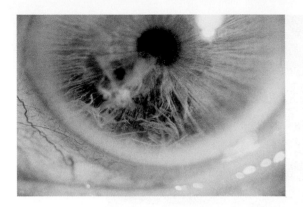

22   Q. Miscellaneous secondary glaucomas – true or false?

a. Approximately 5% of eyes with intraocular tumours develop a secondary elevation of IOP.

b. Melanomalytic glaucoma is due to trabecular blockage by macrophages which have ingested pigment and tumour cells similar to phacolytic glaucoma.

c. Neovascular glaucoma is the most common type in eyes with choroidal melanomas.

d. Most cases of glaucoma in epithelial ingrowth respond well to laser trabeculoplasty.

e. Iridoschisis (see above) typically affects elderly patients and is often bilateral.

f. Ghost cell glaucoma is associated with vitreous haemorrhage.

A.

a. True. **b.** True. **c.** True. **d.** False. **e.** True. **f.** True.

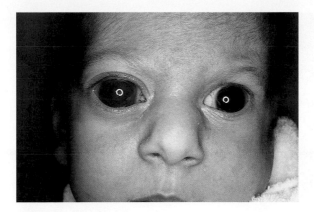

23 Q. Primary congenital glaucoma – answer the following.

a. What is the mode of inheritance?
b. What is the pathogenesis?
c. What is the appearance on gonioscopy?
d. In what percentage of cases is IOP elevated at birth?
e. What is buphthalmos?
f. What are the causes of visual loss?

A.

a. Most cases are sporadic; approximately 10% are AR with incomplete penetrance. **b.** Maldevelopment of the angle of the anterior chamber, unassociated with any other major ocular anomalies (isolated trabeculodysgenesis). **c.** Absence of the ciliary body band due to translucent amorphous material that obscures the trabeculum. **d.** About 40%. **e.** Large eye as a result of stretching due to elevated IOP prior to the age of 3 years (see above). **f.** Optic nerve damage, anisometropic amblyopia, corneal scarring, cataract and lens subluxation.

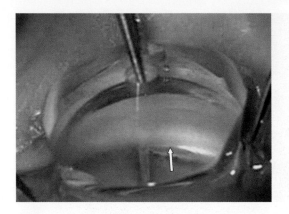

24   Q. Primary congenital glaucoma – true or false?

a. 80% are boys.

b. Corneal haze is the sign most frequently noticed by parents.

c. Corneal diameters of 14 mm are typical of advanced buphthalmos.

d. Haab striae are healed vertical curvilinear lines that represent healed breaks in Descemet membrane.

e. In infants optic cupping may regress when IOP is controlled.

f. Goniotomy (see above) is usually the initial treatment provided the angle can be visualized.

A.

a. False – 65%. **b.** True. **c.** True. **d.** False – horizontal. **e.** True. **f.** True.

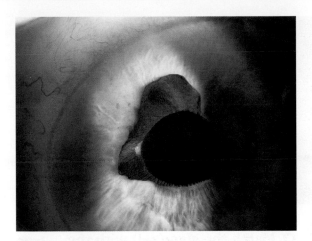

25 Q. Glaucoma in phacomatoses – true or false?

a. Glaucoma develops in about 30% of patients with Sturge–Weber syndrome ipsilateral to the facial haemangioma, especially if the lesion affects the upper eyelid.

b. In Sturge–Weber syndrome eyes with glaucoma often exhibit an episcleral haemangioma.

c. Buphthalmos does not occur in patients with glaucoma and Sturge–Weber syndrome.

d. Glaucoma in Sturge–Weber syndrome is unresponsive to medical treatment.

e. About 50% of patients with neurofibromatosis-1 and glaucoma exhibit either an ipsilateral plexiform neurofibroma of the upper eyelid or exhibit facial hemiatrophy.

f. Glaucoma in neurofibromatosis-1 may be associated with congenital ectropion uveae (see above).

A.

a. True. **b.** True. **c.** False. **d.** False – may respond to topical prostaglandin analogues. **e.** True. **f.** True.

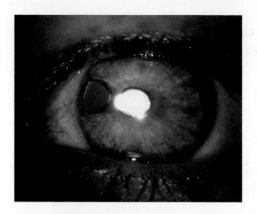

26 Q. Match the sign (a–f) with the appropriate glaucoma (i–vi).

a. Sphincter atrophy.

b. Radial slit-like iris transillumination defects.

c. Glaukomflecken.

d. Iridodonesis.

e. Rubeosis iridis.

f. Pseudopolycoria (see above).

i. Neovascular glaucoma.

ii. Pigmentary glaucoma.

iii. Angle-recession glaucoma.

iv. Acute angle-closure glaucoma.

v. Iridocorneal endothelial syndrome.

vi. Pseudoexfoliation glaucoma.

A.

a. & **vi**; **b.** & **ii**; **c.** & **iv**; **d.** & **iii**; **e.** & **i**; **f.** & **v**.

27 Q. Beta-blockers – answer the following.

a. What is the location of beta-2 receptors?

b. What is the difference between non-selective and cardioselective beta-blockers?

c. How do beta-blockers reduce IOP?

d. What are the main contraindications to beta-blockers?

e. Why should beta-blockers be instilled in the morning and not in the evening?

f. What preparations of timolol are currently available?

A.

a. Bronchi and the ciliary epithelium. **b.** Non-selective are equipotent at beta-1 and beta-2 receptors, while cardioselective are more potent at beta-1 receptors. **c.** By decreasing aqueous secretion. **d.** Congestive cardiac failure, 2nd or 3rd degree heart block, bradycardia, asthma and obstructive airways disease. **e.** Because during sleep, aqueous flow is normally less that half the daytime flow and beta-blockers have little effect. **f.** Timoptol 0.25%, 0.5% b.d., Timoptol-LA 0.25%, 0.5% once daily and Nyogel 0.1% once daily.

28   Q. Beta-blockers – true or false?

a. They may be used in all types of glaucoma.

b. The effect eventually decreases with time in about 20% of patients.

c. When a prostaglandin analogue is added to a beta-blocker a further 20% reduction of IOP occurs.

d. Levobunolol is the only cardioselective beta-blocker currently available.

e. Systemic side-effects usually occur within the first week of administration.

f. Beta-blockers may reduce plasma high-density lipoprotein level.

A.

a. True. **b.** False – effect decreases with time in 10%. **c.** True. **d.** False – betaxolol. **e.** True. **f.** True.

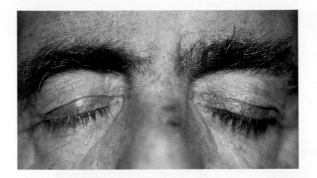

29 Q. Glaucoma medications – answer the following.

a. How do alpha-2 agonists reduce IOP?

b. Why is apraclonidine not suitable for long-term therapy?

c. How does latanoprost lower IOP?

d. Should prostaglandin analogues be instilled in the evening or in the morning?

e. What is the concentration of travoprost?

f. What are the most important adverse effects of prostaglandin analogues?

A.

a. By decreasing aqueous secretion and enhancing uveoscleral outflow.

b. It loses its effect over time (tachyphylaxis) and high incidence of adverse effects. **c.** By increasing uveoscleral outflow. **d.** In the evening. **e.** 0.004%.

f. Lengthening and hyperpigmentation of lashes (see above), and iris pigmentation.

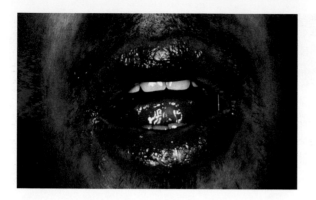

30   Q. Glaucoma medications – true or false?

a. Brimonidine has a neuroprotective effect.

b. Travoprost lowers IOP by enhancing outflow through uveoscleral and trabecular routes.

c. Unoprostone isopropyl 0.15% b.d. is as effective as latanoprost in lowering IOP.

d. Lack of response to latanoprost is rare.

e. Dorzolamide may precipitate corneal endothelial decompensation.

f. Systemic carbonic anhydrase inhibitors may cause Stevens–Johnson syndrome.

A.

a. True. **b.** True. **c.** False – less effective. **d.** False. **e.** True. **f.** True (see above).

31 Q. Match the combined preparation (a–e) with the appropriate constituents (i–v).

a. Cosopt.

b. Xalacom.

c. TimPilo.

d. Combigan.

e. Duotrav.

i. Timolol + brimonidine.

ii. Timolol + latanoprost.

iii. Timolol + dorzolamide.

iv. Timolol + travoprost.

v. Timolol + pilocarpine.

A.

a. & **iii**; **b.** & **ii**; **c.** & **v**; **d.** & **i**; **e.** & **iv**.

32   **Q. Match the glaucoma medication (a–f) with the appropriate side-effect (i–vi).**

a. Oral acetazolamide.

b. Latanoprost.

c. Oral glycerol.

d. Timolol.

e. Pilocarpine.

f. Dorzolamide.

i. Myopia.

ii. Transient bitter taste.

iii. Heterochromia iridis.

iv. Bradycardia.

v. Paraesthesiae.

vi. Urinary retention.

A.

a. & **v**; **b.** & **iii**; **c.** & **vi**; **d.** & **iv**; **e.** & **i**; **f.** & **ii**.

33 Q. Argon laser trabeculoplasty – answer the following.

a. What is argon laser trabeculoplasty?

b. What are the usual initial laser settings?

c. On what part of the trabecular meshwork is the aiming laser beam focused?

d. What is the ideal laser reaction?

e. How many burns are applied to 180° of the trabecular meshwork?

f. What is the initial success rate in POAG?

A.

a. Application of discrete laser burns to the trabecular meshwork to reduce IOP by enhancing aqueous outflow. **b.** 50 μm spot size, 0.1 second duration and 700 mW power. **c.** At the junction of the pigmented and non-pigmented meshwork. **d.** Transient blanching or a minute gas bubble. **e.** 50 burns are applied to 180° of the angle. **f.** 75–85%.

34   Q. Argon laser trabeculoplasty – true or false?

a. It is suitable for paediatric glaucomas provided the angle is open.

b. In cases that fail to show a good response re-treatment is unlikely to be successful once 360° of the trabecular meshwork has been treated.

c. It should never be used as primary treatment.

d. In POAG 50% of eyes are still controlled after 5 years.

e. The results in pseudoexfoliation glaucoma are generally poor.

f. The effect of treatment is usually evident immediately.

A.

a. False. **b.** True. **c.** False. **d.** True. **e.** False – excellent. **f.** False – usually evident within 6 weeks.

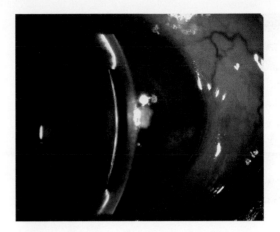

35 Q. Trabeculectomy – answer the following questions.

a. How does trabeculectomy lower IOP?

b. What are the dimensions of the excised deep scleral block?

c. What is the purpose of performing a peripheral iridectomy?

d. What is the purpose of injecting balanced salt solution into the anterior chamber?

e. What is the most common cause of a shallow anterior chamber postoperatively (see above)?

f. What is the pathogenesis of malignant glaucoma?

A.

a. By creating a fistula which allows aqueous outflow from the anterior chamber to the sub-Tenon space. **b.** 1.5 × 2 mm. **c.** To prevent blockage of the internal opening by the iris. **d.** To test the patency of the fistula and to detect any holes or leaks in the conjunctival flap. **e.** Overfiltration.

f. Blockage of aqueous flow at the pars plicata of the ciliary body, so that the aqueous is forced backwards into the vitreous.

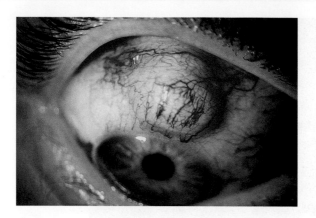

36   Q. Trabeculectomy – true or false?

a. The most common cause of overfiltration is a button hole in the conjunctival flap.

b. Shallow anterior chamber may cause cataract.

c. Initial treatment of malignant glaucoma involves intensive pilocarpine 4%.

d. Encapsulated bleb (Tenon cyst – see above) may develop in the immediate postoperative period.

e. Late bleb leakage may result in maculopathy.

f. Seidel test is negative in overfiltration caused by a bleb leak.

A.

a. False – inadequate closure of the conjunctival flap. **b.** True. **c.** False – intense atropine. **d.** False – 2–8 weeks postoperatively. **e.** True – persistent hypotony. **f.** False.

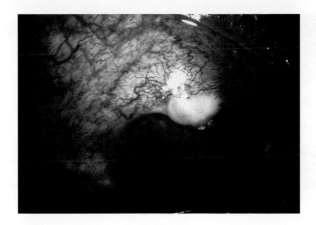

37   Q. Adjunctive antimetabolites – true or false?

a. They inhibit the natural healing response that may preclude successful filtration surgery.

b. They should always be used in most patients with POAG over the age of 70 years.

c. Their most serious complication is blebitis (see above).

d. 5-fluorouracil is an alkylating agent.

e. Mitomycin C is more powerful than 5-fluorouracil.

f. 5-fluorouracil can be injected subconjunctivally in the postoperative period.

A.

a. True. **b.** False. **c.** False – bleb-associated endophthalmitis. **d.** False – antimetabolite. **e.** True. **f.** True.

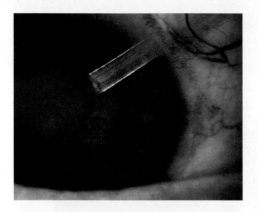

38   Q. Artificial drainage shunts – true or false?

a. They are plastic devices that create a communication between the anterior chamber (see above) and the subconjunctival space.
b. The Molteno implant consists of a silicone tube connected to one or two polypropylene plates 13 mm in diameter.
c. The Ahmed implant consists of a silicone tube connected to a silicone sheet valve held in a polypropylene body.
d. All shunts contain pressure-sensitive valves for regulation of aqueous flow.
e. Adjunctive antimetabolites may enhance the success rate.
f. They should never be used in congenital glaucomas.

A.
a. False – sub-Tenon space. **b.** True. **c.** True. **d.** False. **e.** True. **f.** False.

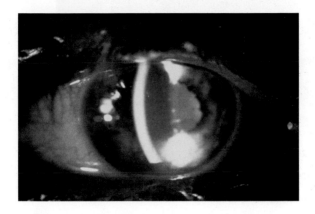

1 **Q. Clinical features – answer the following.**

a. What is the maximal duration of acute anterior uveitis?
b. How is grading of aqueous cells performed?
c. How many cells per field are present in 3+?
d. What is the significance of aqueous flare (see above)?
e. What are the main types of choroiditis?
f. What are the signs of active retinal vasculitis?

A.

a. Up to 3 months. **b.** It is performed with a 2 mm long and 1 mm wide slit beam with maximal light intensity and magnification. **c.** Number of cells per field is 26–50. **d.** Flare reflects the presence of protein due to a break-down of the blood–aqueous barrier **e.** Focal, multifocal and geographic. **f.** Yellowish or grey-white, patchy, perivascular cuffing.

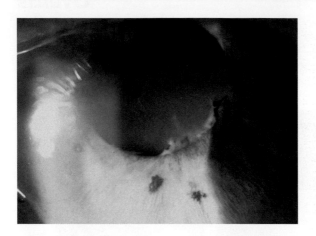

2   Q. Treatment – true or false?

a. Maximal duration of action of atropine is 10 days.

b. Mydricaine consists of a mixture of adrenaline, atropine and procaine.

c. A short-acting mydriatic should be used to prevent the formation of posterior synechiae (see above).

d. Initial dose of ciclosporin is 5 mg/kg/day either as single daily dose or in two divided doses to avoid serum spikes and renal toxicity.

e. Slow-release intraocular steroid implants contain triamcinolone acetonide.

f. Methotrexate should never be used in children.

A.

a. False – up to 2 weeks. **b.** True. **c.** True. **d.** True. **e.** False – fluocinolone acetonide. **f.** False.

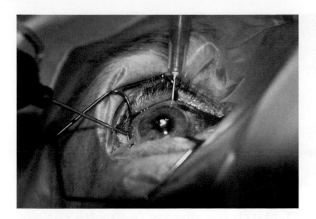

3 Q. The following drugs can be administered intravitreally – true or false?

a. Ganciclovir.

b. Foscarnet.

c. Cidofovir.

d. Dexamethasone.

e. Valaciclovir.

f. Triamcinolone.

A.

a. True. b. True. c. True. d. True. e. False. f. True.

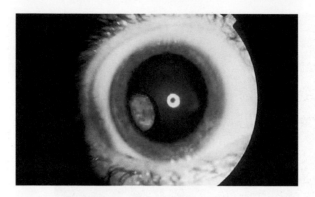

4

Q. Match the disease (a–f) with the appropriate antimicrobial agent (i–vi).

a. Cytomegalovirus retinitis.

b. Acute retinal necrosis.

c. Toxoplasmosis.

d. Cat-scratch disease.

e. Choroidal pneumocystosis.

f. Onchocerciasis.

i. Doxycycline.

ii. Aciclovir.

iii. Vitrasert (see above).

iv. Atovaquone.

v. Trimethoprim.

vi. Ivermectin.

A.

a. & **iii**; b. & **ii**; c. & **iv**; d. & **i**; e. & **v**; f. & **vi**.

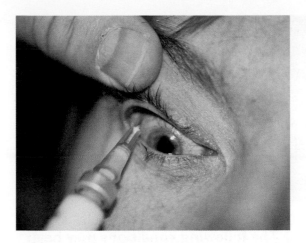

5 Q. Intermediate uveitis – answer the following.

a. What is intermediate uveitis?

b. What is pars planitis?

c. What is the main purpose of performing special investigations?

d. Is the condition most frequently bilateral or unilateral?

e. What is the most common cause of visual impairment?

f. What is the usual initial treatment?

A.

a. An insidious, chronic, relapsing disease in which the vitreous is the major site of the inflammation. **b.** A subset of idiopathic intermediate uveitis in which there is snowbanking or snowball formation. **c.** To detect associated systemic disease. **d.** Usually bilateral but severity of involvement is often asymmetrical. **e.** Chronic cystoid macular oedema. **f.** Posterior sub-Tenon injection of triamcinolone acetonide (see above).

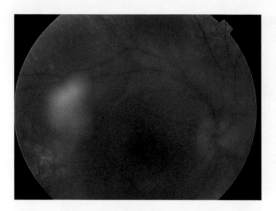

6   **Q. The following conditions may be associated with intermediate uveitis – true or false?**

a. Multiple sclerosis.

b. Juvenile idiopathic arthritis.

c. Lyme disease.

d. Sarcoidosis.

e. Candidiasis.

f. Harada disease.

A.

a. True. **b.** False. **c.** True. **d.** True. **e.** False. **f.** False.

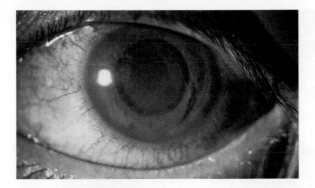

7 Q. Uveitis in spondyloarthropathies – true or false?

a. 10% of men with acute anterior uveitis have ankylosing spondylitis.

b. Anterior uveitis in spondyloarthropathies is frequently associated with a fibrinous exudate (see above).

c. Patients with severe ankylosing spondylitis tend to have more frequent and more severe attacks of acute anterior uveitis.

d. Anterior uveitis in ankylosing spondylitis is always acute.

e. In Reiter disease conjunctivitis is more common than uveitis.

f. Some patients with psoriatic arthritis develop intermediate uveitis.

A.

a. False – 25%. **b.** True. **c.** False – there is no association. **d.** False – some patients develop chronic anterior uveitis. **e.** True. **f.** False.

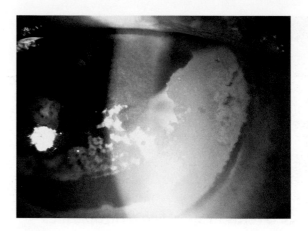

8   Q. Uveitis in idiopathic juvenile idiopathic arthritis (JIA) – answer the following.

a. What are the main risk factors for uveitis in JIA?

b. What is the incidence of uveitis in Still's disease?

c. What are the main characteristics of uveitis?

d. Is there a correlation between activity of arthritis and uveitis?

e. What is the most common cause of permanent visual loss?

f. Can band keratopathy (see above) occur in JIA in the absence of uveitis?

A.

a. Early-onset pauciarticular disease, positive findings for anti-nuclear antibodies and HLA–DR5. **b.** Still's disease is synonymous with systemic-onset JIA which is not associated with uveitis. **c.** It is chronic, non-granulomatous and bilateral in 70% of cases. **d.** No. **e.** Secondary glaucoma. **f.** No.

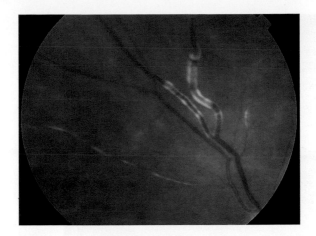

9 Q. Uveitis in bowel disease – true or false?

a. Acute anterior uveitis occurs in about 5% of patients with ulcerative colitis and may synchronize with exacerbation of colitis.
b. Uveitis is more common when ulcerative colitis is associated with ankylosing spondylitis.
c. Chronic anterior uveitis is common in Crohn disease.
d. Periphlebitis (see above) may occur in Crohn disease.
e. Some patients with Crohn disease develop multifocal chorioretinitis.
f. Most patients with Whipple disease do not have uveitis.

A.

a. True. b. True. c. False. d. True. e. False. f. True.

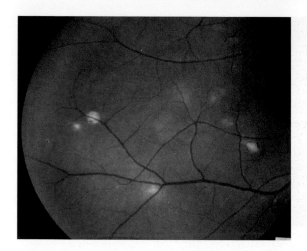

10   **Q. Tubulointerstitial nephritis and uveitis syndrome (TINU) – true or false?**

a. TINU is associated with immunoglobulins depositions in glomerular mesangium.

b. It principally affects young individuals.

c. Renal disease usually precedes uveitis.

d. Mild multifocal choroiditis (see above) occurs in 50% of cases.

e. Anterior uveitis is typically bilateral and non-granulomatous.

f. Anterior uveitis usually responds well to topical steroids.

A.

a. False. **b.** True. **c.** True. **d.** False. **e.** True. **f.** True.

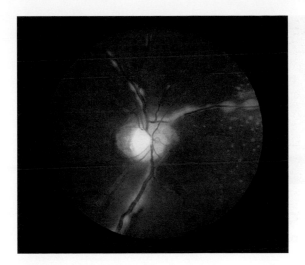

11   Q. Sarcoid uveitis – true or false?

a. Acute anterior uveitis typically affects patients with acute-onset sarcoid.

b. Chronic granulomatous anterior uveitis tends to affect older patients with chronic pulmonary disease.

c. Intermediate uveitis is uncommon and may antedate the onset of systemic disease.

d. Periphlebitis with 'candlewax drippings' (see above) is typical.

e. Multifocal choroiditis may be associated with choroidal neovascularization.

f. Focal granulomas of the optic nerve head usually cause severe visual loss.

A.

a. True. **b.** True. **c.** True. **d.** True. **e.** True. **f.** False.

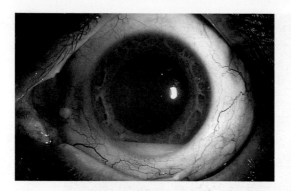

12   Q. Uveitis in Behçet disease – true or false?

a. Uveitis occurs in 70% of men and 95% of women.

b. Uveitis and systemic manifestations usually develop simultaneously.

c. Hypopyon in a quiet eye (see above) is characteristic.

d. Retinal infiltrates may result in severe scarring of the macula.

e. Retinal vasculitis involves veins and arterioles.

f. Systemic steroids are usually adequate as long-term therapy.

A.

a. False – reverse applies. **b.** False. **c.** True. **d.** False – resolve without scarring. **e.** True. **f.** False.

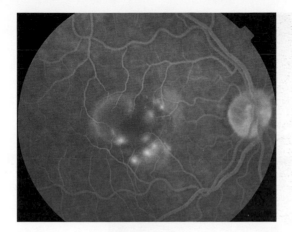

13 Q. Uveitis in Vogt–Koyanagi–Harada syndrome – true or false?

a. Anterior uveitis is granulomatous.

b. Acute posterior segment involvement is characterized by a 'sunset glow' appearance.

c. Fluorescein angiography in the acute stage shows multifocal hyperfluorescent dots at the level of the RPE and the accumulation of dye in the sub-retinal space.

d. Indocyanine green angiography is of no value.

e. Initial treatment involves systemic ciclosporin.

f. Children tend to have a poorer visual prognosis than adults.

A.

a. False – only during recurrences. **b.** False – describes the chronic phase. **c.** True (see above). **d.** False – useful in monitoring the evolution of the choroidal inflammation and the effect of therapy. **e.** False – systemic steroids. **f.** True.

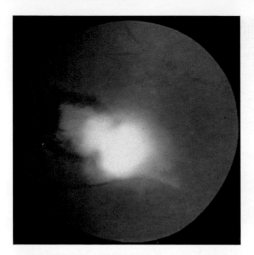

14   Q. Toxoplasma retinitis – true or false?

a. Diagnosis is based on a compatible fundus lesion and positive serology for toxoplasma antibodies irrespective of the titre level.

b. 'Spill-over' anterior uveitis may be granulomatous.

c. Retinitis typically occurs near an old scar.

d. Vitreous cotton-balls are common.

e. Kyrieleis plaques may cause venous occlusion.

f. Choroidal neovascularization may occur adjacent to an old macular scar.

A.

a. True. b. True. c. True (see above). d. False. e. False. f. True.

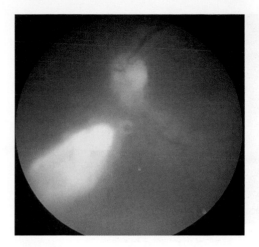

15 Q. Treatment of toxoplasma retinitis – true or false?

a. Not all cases require treatment.

b. Severe vitritis (see above) is not an indication for treatment.

c. There is no evidence to support the benefits of any particular therapeutic regimen.

d. Treatment may cause Stevens–Johnson syndrome.

e. Clindamycin is usually combined with a sulphonamide to prevent pseudomembranous colitis.

f. Pyrimethamine is the drug of choice in patients with AIDS.

A.

a. True. **b.** False. **c.** True. **d.** True – if sulphonamides are used. **e.** True.
f. False – contraindicated.

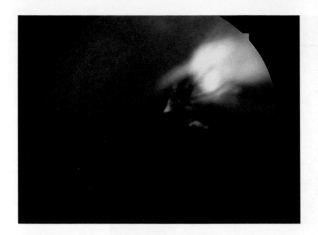

16 Q. Ocular toxocariasis – true or false?

a. Any positive ELISA titre is diagnostic.

b. It is never bilateral.

c. Chronic endophthalmitis presents soon after birth with leukocoria.

d. Differential diagnosis of posterior pole granuloma includes pars planitis.

e. Posterior pole granuloma may cause severe visual loss.

f. Peripheral granuloma (see above) may remain undetected throughout life.

A.

a. False. **b.** True. **c.** False – between the ages of 2 and 9 years. **d.** False – refers to chronic endophthalmitis. **e.** True. **f.** True.

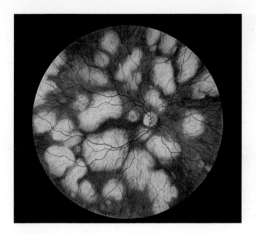

17 Q. Other types of parasitic uveitis – true or false?

a. Anterior uveitis in onchocerciasis may cause miosis.

b. Chorioretinitis in onchocerciasis may resemble 'choroidal sclerosis'.

c. Cysticercosis may cause retinal detachment.

d. Diffuse unilateral subacute neuroretinitis may require argon laser photocoagulation.

e. Choroidal pneumocystosis (see above) occurs in AIDS.

f. Choroidal pneumocystosis has a poor visual prognosis.

A.

a. False – pupil may become pear-shaped. **b.** True. **c.** True. **d.** True.
e. True. **f.** False.

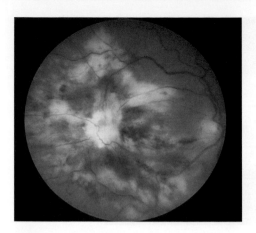

18 **Q. Cytomegalovirus retinitis – true or false?**

a. Since the advent of HAART its incidence has declined and its rate of progression reduced.

b. Indolent retinitis is associated with vasculitis.

c. Fulminating retinitis (see above) is associated with severe vitritis.

d. Side effects of systemic foscarnet include nephrotoxicity, electrolyte disturbances and seizures

e. Intravitreal triamcinolone is useful for indolent chronic cystoid macular oedema.

f. Ganciclovir slow-release device (Vitrasert) has duration of activity of 8 months.

A.

a. True. **b.** False. **c.** False. **d.** True. **e.** False. **f.** True.

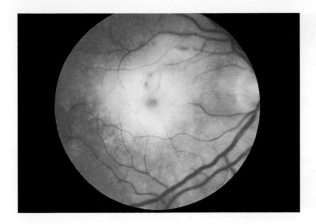

19 Q. Progressive outer retinal necrosis – true or false?

a. Is caused by the varicella zoster virus.

b. It typically affects healthy young men.

c. The name is not appropriate since it is only in the early stages that the infection is limited to the outer retina and there is rapid progression to a full thickness retinal necrosis.

d. Presentation is usually with increasing vitreous floaters due to severe vitritis.

e. Macular involvement is early.

f. Despite early treatment bilateral blindness is the rule.

A.

a. True. **b.** False – it occurs predominantly in AIDS. **c.** True. **d.** False – vitritis is late and mild. **e.** True (see above). **f.** True.

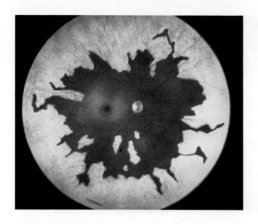

20 Q. Acute retinal necrosis – true or false?

a. Tends to be caused by herpes zoster in younger patients and herpes simplex in older individuals.

b. Typically affects immunosuppressed patients.

c. Anterior granulomatous uveitis and vitritis are universal.

d. Treatment is with systemic aciclovir.

e. Systemic steroids are contraindicated.

f. Visual acuity may be normal in patients with advanced disease.

A.

a. False – reverse applies. **b.** False. **c.** True. **d.** True. **e.** False. **f.** True (see above).

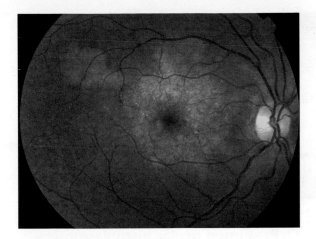

21   Q. Other types of viral uveitis – true or false?

a. Herpes simplex uveitis is always associated with keratitis.

b. Spontaneous hyphaema may occur in herpes simplex uveitis.

c. Anterior uveitis in herpes zoster ophthalmicus is often initially asymptomatic.

d. Elevation of IOP due to trabeculitis may occur in herpes simplex uveitis.

e. Iris atrophy occurs in herpes simplex uveitis but not in herpes zoster uveitis.

f. Rubella retinopathy (see above) is relatively innocuous.

A.

a. False. **b.** True. **c.** True. **d.** True. **e.** False - occurs in both. **f.** True.

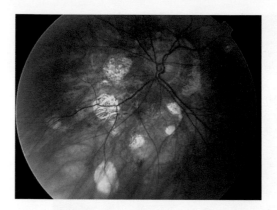

22   Q. Presumed ocular histoplasmosis – true or false?

a. It is associated with an increased prevalence of HLA-B5 and HLA-DR4.

b. Mild granulomatous anterior uveitis is uncommon.

c. 'Histo' spots are scattered in the mid-periphery and posterior fundus.

d. Symptoms are absent in the absence of exudative maculopathy.

e. Choroidal neovascularization occurs in about 50% of eyes.

f. Surgical removal of choroidal neovascular membranes may be appropriate in selected cases.

A.

a. False – HLA-B7 and HLA-DR2. **b.** False – invariably absent. **c.** True (see above). **d.** True. **e.** False – 5%. **f.** True.

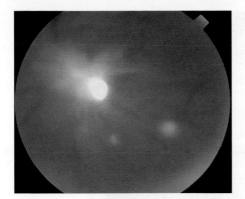

23 Q. Endogenous fungal endophthalmitis
– true or false?

a. Intravenous drug abuse is a common predisposition.

b. *Candida* spp. are frequent pathogens.

c. Progression is faster than in bacterial endophthalmitis.

d. Bilateral involvement is rare.

e. Pars plana vitrectomy may be required if vitreous involvement is severe (see above).

f. Systemic steroids should be used in severe cases.

A.

a. True. **b.** True. **c.** False – slower. **d.** False – common. **e.** True. **f.** False.

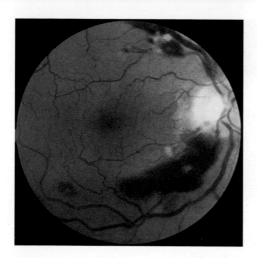

24   **Q. Endogenous (metastatic) endophthalmitis – true or false?**

a. The most common pathogen is *Pseudomonas aeruginosa.*

b. Initial misdiagnosis is common.

c. Anterior uveitis is absent.

d. Roth spots (see above) are characteristic.

e. All patients require blood cultures.

f. Mortality from associated systemic disease is 5–10%.

A.

a. False – *Klebsiella* spp. **b.** True. **c.** False. **d.** False. **e.** True. **f.** True.

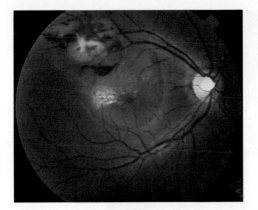

25   Q. Tuberculous uveitis – true or false?

a. May occur in the absence of systemic manifestations.

b. Chronic anterior uveitis is the most common feature.

c. Choroiditis is caused by a hypersensitivity to the bacillus.

d. Choroiditis may resemble serpiginous choroidopathy.

e. Periphlebitis may be occlusive (see above).

f. Large solitary granulomas are common.

A.

a. True. **b.** True. **c.** False – direct infection. **d.** True. **e.** True. **f.** False.

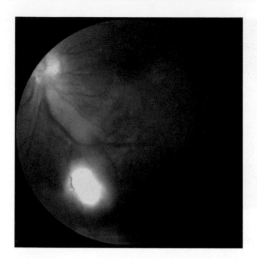

26   Q. Syphilitic uveitis – true or false?

a. It is a common cause of uveitis in AIDS.

b. Typically occurs during the primary stage.

c. Anterior uveitis is bilateral in 50% of cases.

d. Focal chorioretinitis (see above) is more common than multifocal.

e. Neuroretinitis frequently leads to optic atrophy.

f. Treatment with conventional doses of penicillin is adequate.

A.

a. False. **b.** False – secondary and tertiary stages. **c.** True. **d.** False – reverse applies. **e.** True. **f.** False.

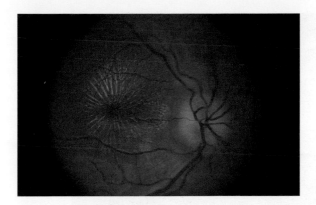

27 Q. Other types of bacterial uveitis – true or false?

a. Uveitis is uncommon in Lyme disease.

b. Uveitis in Lyme disease is treated with systemic doxycycline and rifampicin.

c. Intermediate uveitis does not occur in brucellosis.

d. Neuroretinitis (see above) is the most common ocular manifestation of cat-scratch disease.

e. In neuroretinitis both macular exudates and papillitis resolve simultaneously.

f. Iris pearls are pathognomonic for lepromatous iritis.

A.

a. True. **b.** False – topical steroids. **c.** True. **d.** True. **e.** False – exudates may worsen as papillitis resolves. **f.** True.

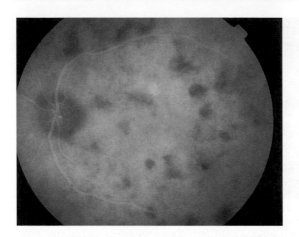

28 **Q. Acute posterior multifocal placoid pigment epitheliopathy – true or false?**

a. It is associated with HLA-B7 and HLA-DR2.

b. It is more common in males.

c. Some patients have an associated flu-like illness.

d. Treatment is with systemic steroids.

e. Choroidal neovascularization develops in 10% of cases.

f. Indocyanine green angiography is superior to fluorescein angiography in demonstrating non-perfusion of the choriocapillaris.

A.

a. True. b. False – both sexes are equally affected. c. True. d. False.
e. False. f. True (see above).

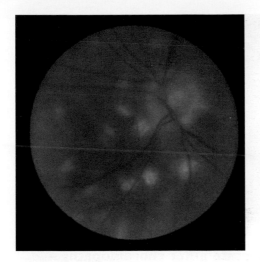

29 Q. Birdshot retinochoroidopathy – true or false?

a. Typically affects young adults.

b. Night blindness may be the presenting symptom.

c. Severe vitritis with snow-balls is common.

d. It is characterized by multiple, small, ill-defined, cream-coloured, choroidal spots in the posterior pole and mid-periphery.

e. Fluorescein angiography shows more lesions than are apparent clinically.

f. The decision to treat is based on ERG findings.

A.

a. False – fifth to seventh decades. **b.** True. **c.** False – vitritis is mild and snow-balls absent. **d.** True (see above). **e.** False – reverse applies.
f. True.

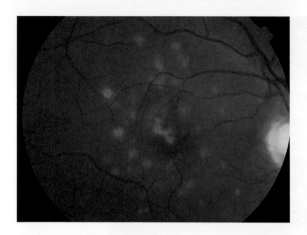

30   Q. Punctate inner choroidopathy – true or false?

a. Typically affects young myopic women.

b. Anterior uveitis is severe.

c. The lesions are all of the same age and principally involve the posterior pole.

d. Treatment is with ciclosporin and systemic steroids.

e. CNV (type 2 – under the sensory retina) develops in up to 40% of patients.

f. ERG is normal.

A.

a. True. **b.** False – is absent. **c.** True (see above). **d.** False. **e.** True.
f. True.

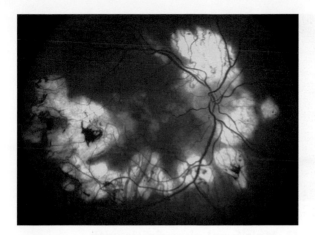

31   Q. Serpiginous choroidopathy – true or false?

a. It affects men more than women and is associated with HLA-B7.

b. Involvement is usually unilateral.

c. It may be inactive for prolonged periods before recurring.

d. Inactive lesions are characterized by scalloped, atrophic, 'punched-out' areas of choroidal and RPE atrophy.

e. Subretinal fibrosis is a common complication.

f. Prognosis is poor and 50–75% of patients will eventually develop visual loss.

A.

a. True. **b.** False. **c.** True. **d.** True (see above). **e.** False. **f.** True.

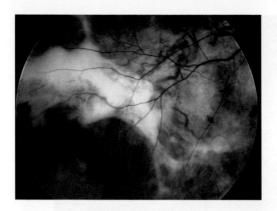

32   Q. Multifocal choroiditis with panuveitis – true or false?

a. It typically affects middle-aged women.

b. Chronic anterior uveitis is universal.

c. In older patients the lesions may be confined to the periphery.

d. Inactive lesions may resemble presumed ocular histoplasmosis.

e. It is unresponsive to steroids.

f. Subretinal fibrosis (see above) is common in end-stage disease.

A.

a. True. **b.** False – in 50%. **c.** True. **d.** True. **e.** False – effective if administered early. **f.** False – rare.

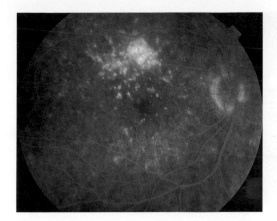

33 Q. Multiple evanescent white dot syndrome – true or false?

a. Most cases are bilateral.

b. An afferent pupillary defect may be present.

c. It is characterized by numerous, very small, ill-defined, white dots involving the mid-periphery and macula.

d. Physiological blind spot may be enlarged.

e. Fluorescein angiography shows numerous hypofluorescent spots.

f. Treatment is not required.

A.

a. False – unilateral. **b.** True. **c.** False – macula is spared. **d.** True.

e. False – hyperfluorescent (see above). **f.** True.

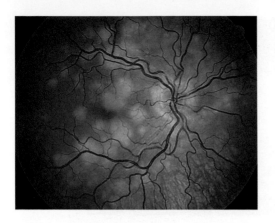

34 **Q. The following may be associated with choroidal neovascularization – true or false?**

a. Multifocal choroiditis with panuveitis.

b. Punctate inner choroidopathy.

c. Multiple evanescent white dot syndrome.

d. Acute retinal pigment epitheliitis.

e. Acute multifocal posterior placoid pigment epitheliopathy (see above).

f. Serpiginous choroidopathy.

A.

a. True. b. True. c. False. d. False. e. False. f. True.

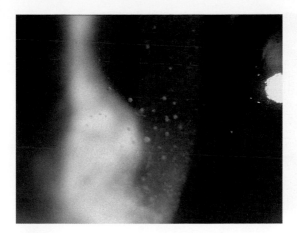

35 Q. Fuchs uveitis syndrome – true or false?

a. Heterochromia iridis is the most common presenting finding.

b. Posterior synechiae develop in longstanding cases.

c. Keratic precipitates are small and scattered throughout the endothelium.

d. Iris nodules may be present.

e. Treatment involves topical steroids and mydriatics.

f. Secondary glaucoma is a late feature.

A.

a. False. **b.** False – invariably absent. **c.** True (see above). **d.** True.
e. False. **f.** True.

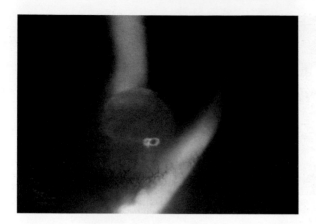

36   Q. Lens-induced uveitis – true or false?

a. Is triggered by an immune response to lens proteins following rupture of the lens capsule.

b. Phacoanaphylactic endophthalmitis eventually becomes bilateral.

c. Phacoanaphylactic endophthalmitis is often associated with elevation of IOP.

d. Phacoanaphylactic endophthalmitis is confined to the anterior segment.

e. Phacogenic non-granulomatous uveitis develops within 1 week of capsular rupture.

f. Phacogenic non-granulomatous uveitis is chronic.

A.

a. True (see above – residual lens material in the anterior chamber).

b. False. **c.** True. **d.** True. **e.** False – 2–3 weeks. **f.** True.

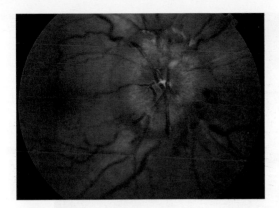

37 Q. Match (a–f) with the appropriate micro-organism (i–vi).

a. Choroidal neovascularization.

b. Iris pearls.

c. Pear-shaped pupil.

d. Chronic endophthalmitis.

e. Neuroretinitis.

f. Papilloedema (see above).

i. *Cryptococcus neoformans.*

ii. *Bartonella henselae.*

iii. *Candida albicans.*

iv. *Histoplasma capsulatum.*

v. *Mycobacterium leprae.*

vi. *Onchocerca volvulus.*

A.

a. & **iv**; b. & **v**; c. & **vi**; d. & **iii**; e. & **ii**; f. & **i**.

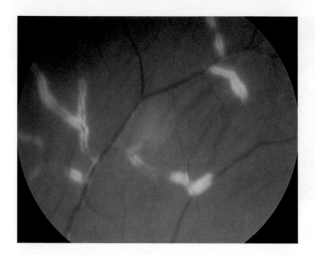

38   Q. Retinal vasculitis – true or false?

a. Most cases are idiopathic.

b. It may occur in intermediate uveitis.

c. Frosted branch angiitis (see above) may be associated with infectious retinitis.

d. In sarcoidosis it may be associated with candlewax perivenous exudates.

e. In Behçet disease it involves only arteries.

f. In multiple sclerosis it is usually asymptomatic.

A.

a. False. b. True. c. True. d. True. e. False – both vein and arteries.
f. True.

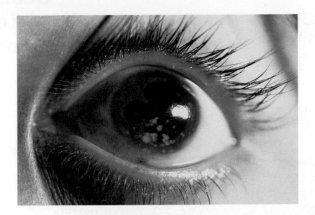

39 Q. The following are associated with granulomatous anterior uveitis – true or false?

a. Vogt–Koyanagi–Harada syndrome.

b. Behçet disease.

c. Juvenile idiopathic arthritis.

d. Sarcoidosis.

e. Toxoplasmosis.

f. Wegener granulomatosis.

A.

a. True. b. False. c. False. d. True e. True. f. False.

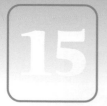

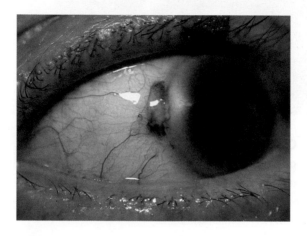

1 Q. Conjunctival naevus – true or false?

a. Is more common in black individuals.

b. Presentation is during the first 2 decades of life.

c. Junctional naevi are more common than compound.

d. The most common location is juxtalimbal.

e. After puberty it may become less pigmented.

f. Cystic spaces may indicate malignant transformation.

A.

a. False. **b.** True. **c.** False – reverse applies. **d.** True (see above).

e. False – more pigmented. **f.** False.

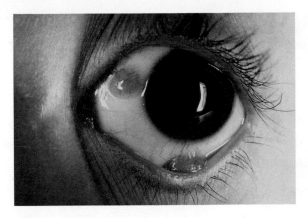

2 Q. Conjunctival papilloma – true or false?

a. Pedunculated papillomas (see above) are caused by human papillomavirus.

b. Pedunculated papillomas may present in infancy.

c. Recurrent pedunculated papillomas may require topical mitomycin.

d. Sessile papillomas usually present in middle-age.

e. Sessile papillomas may be multiple and bilateral.

f. Sessile papillomas are treated by cryotherapy.

A.

a. True. **b.** True. **c.** True. **d.** True. **e.** False – applies to pedunculated lesions. **f.** False.

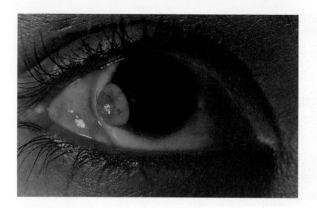

3   Q. Epibulbar choristoma – true or false?

a. Choristoma is a congenital overgrowth of normal tissue in an abnormal location.

b. Solid dermoids are most frequently located at the nasal limbus.

c. Solid dermoids typically develop in puberty.

d. Solid dermoids may be associated with Goldenhar syndrome.

e. Lipodermoids are most frequently located at the outer canthus.

f. Lipodermoids should be excised.

A.

a. True. **b.** False – temporal (see above). **c.** False – early childhood.

d. True. **e.** True. **f.** False – treatment should be avoided.

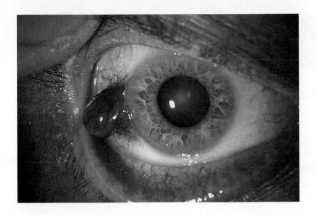

4 Q. Conjunctival melanoma – true or false?

a. Accounts for about 2% of all ocular malignancies.

b. The majority of cases arise from primary acquired melanosis with atypia.

c. It never arises from a pre-existing naevus.

d. Primary melanoma is never amelanotic.

e. The limbus is a common location of primary melanoma.

f. Exenteration for orbital recurrences does not improve the prognosis for life.

A.

a. True. **b.** True. **c.** False – about 20% arise from pre-existing naevi.
d. False. **e.** True (see above). **f.** True.

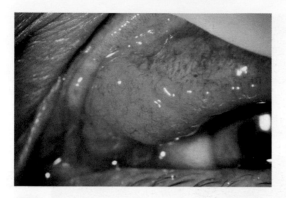

5   Q. Other conjunctival tumours – true or false?

a. Xeroderma pigmentosum is a risk factor for conjunctival intraepithelial neoplasia.

b. Histology of carcinoma *in situ* shows dysplastic cells in the basal layers of the epithelium.

c. Squamous cell carcinoma frequently metastasises.

d. Most conjunctival lymphomas (see above) are B cell lymphomas and arise from MALT.

e. Most conjunctival lymphomas are associated with systemic involvement.

f. Kaposi sarcoma may mimic a subconjunctival haemorrhage.

A.

a. True. **b.** False – dysplastic cells involve the full thickness of the epithelium. **c.** False – metastatic spread is rare. **d.** True. **e.** False. **f.** True.

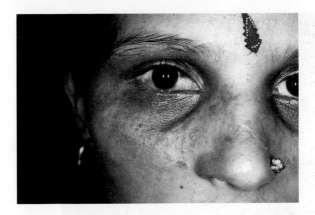

6   Q. The following conditions predispose to uveal melanoma – true or false?

a. Light iris colour.

b. Familial cutaneous melanoma.

c. Naevus of Ota (see above).

d. Uveal melanocytoma.

e. Gorlin–Goltz syndrome.

f. Neurofibromatosis-1.

A.

a. True. b. True. c. True. d. True. e. False. f. True.

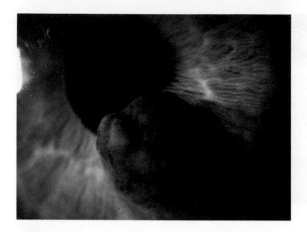

7   Q. Iris tumours – true or false?

a. Typical iris naevus is less than 3 mm in diameter.

b. Diffuse iris naevus may be associated with glaucoma.

c. The majority of iris melanomas involve the superior half of the iris.

d. Most iris melanomas are composed of spindle cells.

e. Iris melanomas present later than choroidal melanomas.

f. Iris melanomas may be associated with severe anterior uveitis.

A.

a. True. b. True – in the context of Cogan–Reese syndrome. c. False – inferior half (see above). d. True. e. False – earlier. f. False.

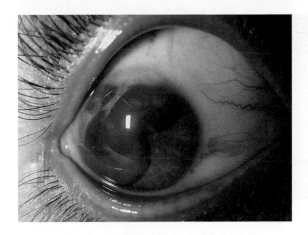

8   Q. Iris cysts – true or false?

a. Primary epithelial cysts are often multiple.

b. Primary epithelial cysts may dislodge into the anterior chamber.

c. Primary stromal cysts develop in puberty.

d. Most primary stromal cysts eventually require treatment.

e. Most secondary cysts occur following surgery or penetrating trauma.

f. Long-acting miotics may cause bilateral secondary cysts.

A.

a. False – solitary. **b.** True. **c.** False – early childhood. **d.** True. **e.** True.

f. True (see above).

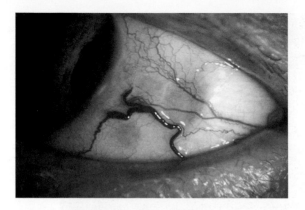

9   Q. Ciliary body melanoma – true or false?

a. Comprises 15% of uveal melanomas.

b. May mimic both an iris melanoma and a conjunctival melanoma.

c. May be asymptomatic and discovered by chance.

d. Sentinel vessels (see above) imply extraocular extension.

e. Should be considered in the differential diagnosis of exudative retinal detachment.

f. Radiotherapy is not appropriate.

A.

a. False – 5%. **b.** True. **c.** True. **d.** False. **e.** True. **f.** False.

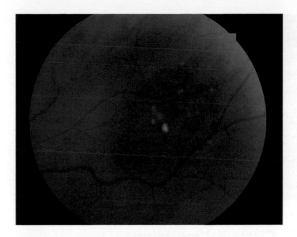

10   Q. Choroidal naevus – true or false?

a. Is rare in non-caucasians.

b. Histology shows proliferation of spindle cells in the choriocapillaris.

c. It is characterized by a grey oval lesion with sharp borders.

d. Fluorescein is helpful in distinguishing a naevus from a small melanoma.

e. Surface lipofuscin is common on large naevi.

f. The vast majority do not require follow-up.

A.

a. True. **b.** False – choriocapillaris is spared. **c.** False – not sharp (see above). **d.** False. **e.** False – lipofuscin is characteristic of melanoma. **f.** True.

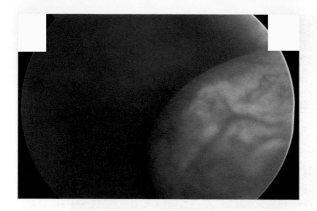

11   Q. Choroidal melanoma – true or false?

a. Accounts for 50% of uveal melanomas.

b. The main histological types are spindle cell and necrotic.

c. Amelanotic tumours (see above) are common.

d. Fluorescein angiography should be performed in most cases.

e. Enucleation is the most frequent treatment.

f. External radiotherapy and brachytherapy are equally effective in selected cases.

A.

a. False – 85%. **b.** False – epithelioid cell. **c.** True. **d.** False. **e.** False.
f. True.

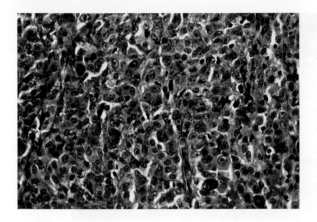

12 **Q. The following are unfavourable prognostic factors in choroidal melanoma – true or false?**

a. Large tumour.

b. Macular involvement.

c. Presentation in the eighth decade.

d. Collar-stud shape.

e. Histology showing a large number of epithelioid cells.

f. Cytogenetic abnormalities such as gains in chromosome 8.

A.

a. True. b. False. c. True. d. False. e. True (see above). f. True.

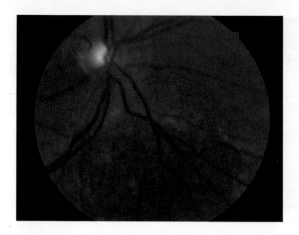

13   **Q. The following should be considered in the differential diagnosis of choroidal melanoma – true or false?**

a. Intraocular lymphoma.

b. Melanocytoma.

c. Choroidal osteoma.

d. Exudative retinal detachment.

e. Large melanocytic lesions touching the disc.

f. Choroidal metastasis.

A.

a. False. **b.** True. **c.** False. **d.** True. **e.** True (see above). **f.** True.

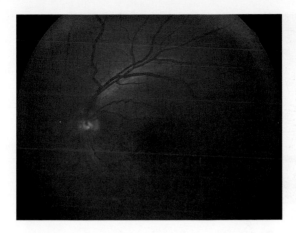

14 Q. Choroidal haemangioma – true or false?

a. May remain dormant throughout life.

b. Most do not involve the macula.

c. Fluorescein angiography shows rapid, spotty hyperfluorescence in the prearterial or early arterial phase and diffuse intense late hyperfluorescence.

d. Photodynamic therapy may be appropriate in circumscribed tumours.

e. Diffuse tumours (see above) are treated with brachytherapy.

f. Patients with diffuse lesions may have ipsilateral naevus flammeus.

A.

a. True. **b.** False. **c.** True. **d.** True. **e.** False – external beam radiotherapy. **f.** True.

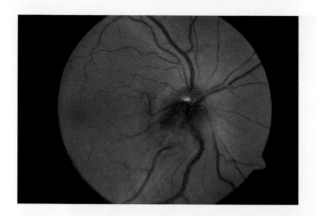

15   Q. Optic nerve head melanocytoma – true or false?

a. It typically affects dark-skinned females.

b. It usually grows throughout life.

c. Early treatment is required to prevent malignant transformation.

d. May cause retinal vein occlusion.

e. Afferent pupillary defect may be seen even when vision is normal.

f. Special investigations are not required for diagnosis.

A.

a. True. **b.** False – most are stationary. **c.** False – malignant transformation is very rare. **d.** True. **e.** True. **f.** True.

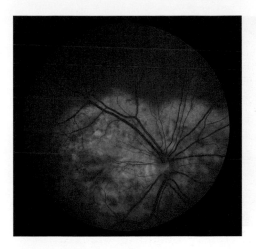

16 Q. Osseous choristoma (choroidal osteoma) – true or false?

a. It typically affects females.

b. It is bilateral in 25% of cases.

c. Presentation is in old age.

d. It is characterized by an orange-yellow lesion with well-defined, scalloped borders near the disc or at the posterior pole.

e. Choroidal vascularization may cause visual loss.

f. MR demonstrates bone-like features.

A.

a. True. **b.** True. **c.** False – second to third decades. **d.** True (see above). **e.** True. **f.** False – MR does not show bone.

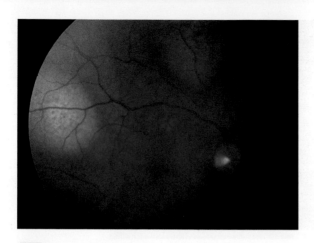

17 Q. Metastatic choroidal tumours – true or false?

a. Bronchus is a rare primary site in women.

b. Prostate is a common primary site in men.

c. Deposits are multifocal (see above) in about 30% of patients and bilateral in 10–30%.

d. Secondary exudative retinal detachment occurs only if the tumour is large.

e. Fluorescein angiography shows early hypofluorescence and diffuse late staining but a 'dual circulation' is not seen.

f. Systemic therapy for the primary tumour does not influence the choroidal deposits.

A.

a. False. **b.** False. **c.** True. **d.** False. **e.** True. **f.** False.

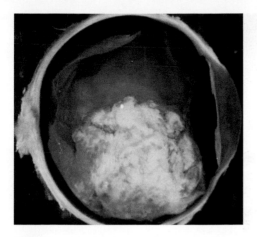

18 Q. Retinoblastoma – answer the following.

a. What is the most common presenting feature?
b. What is the average age at presentation of unilateral cases?
c. What are endophytic and exophytic growth patterns?
d. Which systemic cytotoxic drugs may be used in chemotherapy?
e. What is chemoreduction?
f. Why should external beam radiotherapy be avoided in patients with heritable tumours?

A.

a. Leukocoria. **b.** 2 years of age. **c.** Endophytic growth is into the vitreous (see above) and exophytic into the sub-retinal space.
d. Carboplatin, vincristine and etoposide. **e.** Chemotherapy to shrink the tumour and facilitate subsequent local treatment. **f.** Because of the risk of inducing a second malignancy such as osteosarcoma.

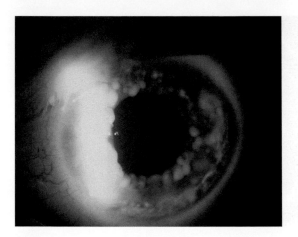

19   Q. Retinoblastoma – true or false?

a. It accounts for a small minority of all childhood cancers.

b. Heritable (germline) retinoblastoma accounts for 60% of cases.

c. If a child has heritable retinoblastoma, the risk to siblings is 2% if the parents are healthy, and 40% if a parent is affected.

d. Retinoblastoma in older children may mimic anterior uveitis.

e. Orbital signs invariably indicate extraocular extension.

f. Treatment of most large unilateral tumours involves enucleation.

A.

a. True – 3%. **b.** False – 40%. **c.** True. **d.** True (see above). **e.** False.
f. False.

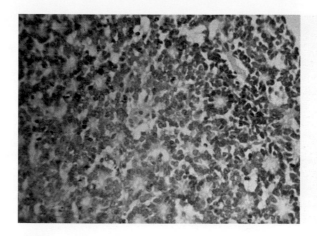

20   Q. The following are unfavourable prognostic factors in retinoblastoma – true or false?

a. Optic nerve involvement.

b. Large tumour.

c. Extensive choroidal invasion.

d. Abundant Flexner–Wintersteiner rosettes (see above).

e. Orbital inflammation.

f. Heritable case.

A.

a. True. **b.** True. **c.** True. **d.** False – implies well-differentiated tumour.

e. False – does not necessarily imply orbital invasion. **f.** False.

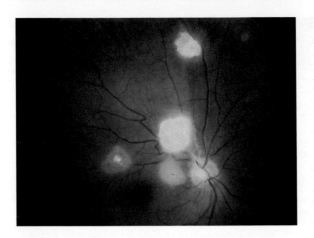

21   Q. Astrocytoma – true or false?

a. It does not usually threaten vision.

b. It occurs exclusively in patients with tuberous-sclerosis.

c. About 50% of patients with tuberous sclerosis have astrocytomas which may be multiple (see above).

d. Most exhibit very slow growth.

e. Most involve the optic nerve head.

f. Fluorescein shows autofluorescence and hyperfluorescence due to staining without leakage.

A.

a. True. **b.** False. **c.** True. **d.** False. **e.** False. **f.** True.

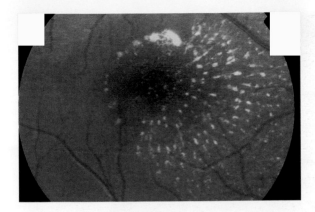

22   Q. Retinal haemangioblastoma – true or false?

a. About 60% of patients with multiple tumours have von Hippel–Lindau disease.

b. Is usually endophytic and occasionally exophytic.

c. Age at presentation is earlier in patients without associated von Hippel–Lindau disease.

d. A macular star (see above) may be seen in eyes with peripheral tumours.

e. All peripheral tumours should be treated.

f. Photodynamic therapy may be appropriate for juxtapapillary tumours.

A.

a. False – virtually all patients with multiple tumours have von Hippel–Lindau disease. **b.** True. **c.** False. **d.** True. **e.** True. **f.** True.

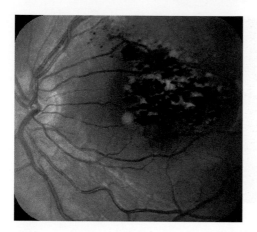

23 Q. Other retinal vascular tumours – true or false?

a. Cavernous haemangioma are often associated with lesions of the skin and brain.

b. Cavernous haemangiomas (see above) require early treatment to prevent vitreous haemorrhage.

c. Racemose haemangioma resembles a cluster of grapes.

d. Some patients with racemose haemangioma develop cerebral haemorrhage.

e. Fluorescein in racemose haemangioma shows early hyperfluorescence and late leakage.

f. Vasoproliferative tumour may occur in intermediate uveitis.

A.

a. False – association is rare. **b.** False – most are innocuous. **c.** False – applies to cavernous haemangioma. **d.** True – only if they have Wyburn–Mason syndrome. **e.** False – leakage is absent. **f.** True.

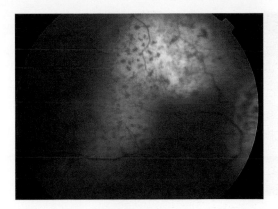

24   Q. Primary intraocular lymphoma – true or false?

a. It represents a subset of primary central nervous system lymphoma which is a variant of extranodal non-Hodgkin lymphoma.

b. Onset is in middle-age.

c. Vitreous 'snowballs' are common.

d. Multifocal sub-RPE infiltration may resemble amelanotic melanoma.

e. Vitreous biopsy shows large, malignant lymphocytes with irregular nuclei, prominent nucleoli and scanty cytoplasm.

f. Intravitreal methotrexate is useful for recurrent disease.

A.

a. True. **b.** False – old age. **c.** False – vitreous sheets. **d.** False (see above). **e.** True. **f.** True.

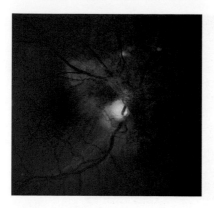

25   Q. Tumours of the retinal pigment epithelium RPE – true or false?

a. Congenital hypertrophy of the RPE is frequently juxtapapillary.

b. In 'bear-track' pigmentation the smaller lesions are usually more peripheral.

c. Some patients with atypical congenital hypertrophy of the RPE develop carcinoma of the colon.

d. Combined hamartoma of the retina and RPE may cause 'dragging' of the disc and macula.

e. Combined hamartoma of the retina and RPE responds well to vitreoretinal surgery if performed early.

f. Congenital hamartoma of the RPE is usually asymptomatic.

A.

a. False. **b.** False. **c.** True. **d.** True. **e.** False. **f.** True.

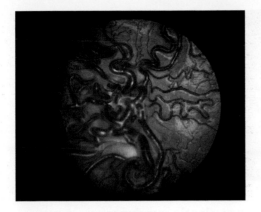

26 Q. Match the fundus lesion (a–f) with the appropriate systemic condition (i–vi).

a. Capillary haemangioblastoma.

b. Astrocytoma.

c. Racemose haemangioma
(see above).

d. Congenital hypertrophy of RPE.

e. Diffuse choroidal haemangioma.

f. Choroidal melanoma.

i. Gardner syndrome.

ii. Bourneville syndrome.

iii. Wyburn–Mason
syndrome.

iv. von Hippel–Lindau
syndrome.

v. Naevus of Ota.

vi. Sturge–Weber syndrome.

A.

a. & **iv**; b. & **ii**; c. & **iii**; d. & **i**; e. & **vi**; f. & **v**.

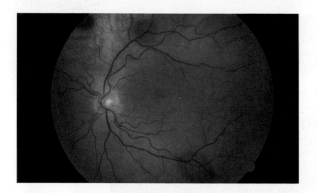

27   Q. Paraneoplastic syndromes – true or false?

a. In bilateral diffuse melanocytic proliferation (see above) treatment of the tumour may result in visual improvement.

b. Bilateral diffuse uveal melanocytic proliferation may be associated with choroidal neovascularization.

c. Cancer-associated retinopathy is most frequently associated with small-cell bronchial carcinoma.

d. In cancer-associated retinopathy the ERG is severely attenuated under photopic and scotopic conditions.

e. Melanoma-associated retinopathy presents with gradual, peripheral visual-field loss.

f. Melanoma-associated retinopathy has a good visual prognosis.

A.

a. False. **b.** False. **c.** True. **d.** True. **e.** False – visual loss is sudden and central. **f.** True.

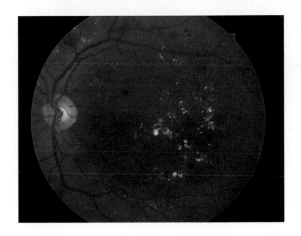

1   Q. Diabetic retinopathy – true or false?

a. It is more common in type 1 than in type 2 diabetes.

b. Poor metabolic control is the most important risk factor.

c. It rarely develops before puberty.

d. About 5% of type 2 diabetics have retinopathy (see above) at presentation.

e. Raised HbA1c is associated with an increased risk of maculopathy.

f. Tight control of hypertension appears to be particularly beneficial in type 1 diabetics with proliferative disease.

A.

a. True. **b.** False – duration of diabetes. **c.** True. **d.** True. **e.** False – proliferative disease. **f.** False – type 2 diabetics with maculopathy.

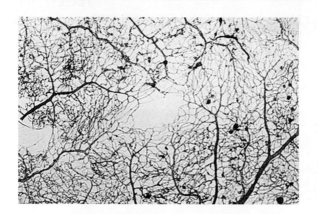

2   Q. Histological changes in diabetic retinopathy – true or false?

a. Thickening of the capillary basement membrane.

b. Proliferation of pericytes.

c. Loss of endothelial cells.

d. Microaneurysms.

e. Capillary closure.

f. Arteriolosclerosis.

A.

a. True. **b.** False – loss. **c.** False – proliferation. **d.** True (see above).
e. True. **f.** False.

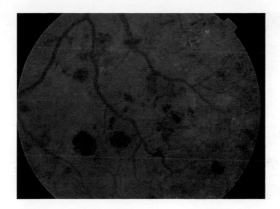

**Q. Background diabetic retinopathy –
answer the following.**

a. What are the earliest findings?

b. What is the pathogenesis and composition of hard exudates?

c. What is the location of hard exudates within the retina?

d. What is the pathogenesis of localized retinal oedema?

e. Why do intraretinal haemorrhages have a 'dot-blot'
configuration (see above)?

f. What is the treatment of simple background diabetic
retinopathy?

A.

a. Microaneurysms. **b.** Hard exudates are caused by chronic localized
retinal oedema and develop at the junction of normal and oedematous
retina. They are composed of lipoprotein and lipid-filled macrophages.
c. Outer plexiform layer. **d.** Focal leakage from microaneurysms and
dilated capillary segments. **e.** Because an end-on view is seen as they
are located within the compact middle layers of the retina. **f.** Treatment
is not required.

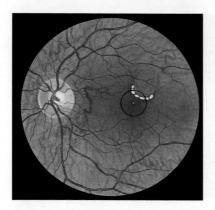

 Q. Signs of clinically significant macular oedema – true or false?

a. Retinal oedema within 500 µm of the centre of the fovea.

b. Hard exudates within 500 µm of the fovea if associated with retinal thickening.

c. Cystoid macular oedema.

d. Dot-blot haemorrhages within 500 µm of the centre of the fovea.

e. Retinal oedema that is one disc area or larger, any part of which is within one disc diameter of the centre of the fovea.

f. Area of non-perfusion seen on fluorescein angiography within 500 µm of the centre of the fovea.

A.

a. True. **b.** True (see above). **c.** False. **d.** False. **e.** True. **f.** False.

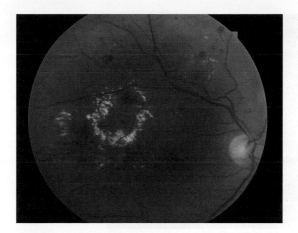

5   Q. Diabetic maculopathy – true or false?

a. It is the most common cause of visual loss in diabetics.

b. Focal maculopathy is characterized by well-circumscribed retinal thickening associated with rings of hard exudates.

c. Eyes with diffuse maculopathy frequently show peripheral non-perfusion on fluorescein angiography.

d. Ischaemic maculopathy may respond to intravitreal triamcinolone acetonide.

e. Visual improvement occurs in 15% of eyes following grid treatment for diffuse diabetic maculopathy.

f. Laser therapy for clinically significant macular oedema reduces the risk of visual loss by 50%.

A.

a. True. **b.** True (see above). **c.** False – applies to ischaemic maculopathy.
d. False – applies to diffuse maculopathy. **e.** True. **f.** True.

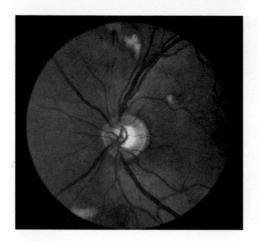

6   Q. The following occur in pre-proliferative diabetic retinopathy – true or false?

a. Cotton-wool spots (see above).

b. Severe macular oedema.

c. Venous tortuosity.

d. Peripheral neovascularization.

e. Intraretinal microvascular abnormalities.

f. Dark-blot haemorrhages.

A.

a. True. **b.** False. **c.** True. **d.** False. **e.** True. **f.** True.

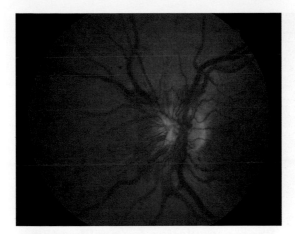

7 **Q. Proliferative diabetic retinopathy – answer the following.**

a. What is the incidence in type 1 diabetics after 30 years?
b. What are the criteria for mild and severe disc vessels?
c. What is the risk of severe visual loss within 2 years of untreated eyes with severe disc new vessels and haemorrhage?
d. What is the most serious complication?
e. What is the usual initial spot size and duration of a laser burn when performing panretinal laser photocoagulation with a Goldmann lens?
f. What are signs of evolution following successful laser therapy?

A.

a. About 60%. **b.** Mild when less than one-third disc area is covered by new vessels; severe when more than one-third disc area is covered (see above). **c.** 30%. **d.** Tractional retinal detachment involving the macula. **e.** Spot size 200–500 μm and duration 0.1–0.2 seconds. **f.** Regression of neovascularization leaving 'ghost' vessels or fibrous tissue, decrease in venous changes, absorption of retinal haemorrhages and disc pallor.

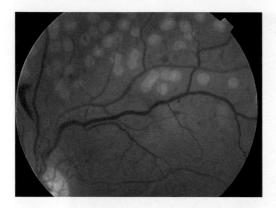

8 **Q. Photocoagulation for proliferative diabetic retinopathy – true or false?**

a. All eyes require urgent treatment.

b. Fluorescein angiography is required prior to treatment.

c. Treatment should be completed in one session.

d. Low-intensity burns (see above) are adequate.

e. Recurrences may occur despite an initial satisfactory response.

f. A response is usually evident within 2 weeks.

A.

a. False – only high-risk cases. **b.** False. **c.** False. **d.** True. **e.** True. **f.** False – 4–6 weeks.

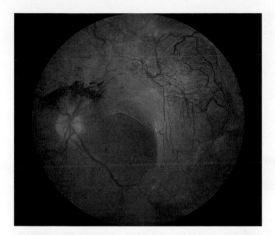

9 **Q. The following are indications for pars plana vitrectomy in diabetic eye disease – true or false?**

a. All tractional retinal detachments.

b. Progressive tractional retinal detachment threatening or involving the macula.

c. Combined tractional and rhegmatogenous retinal detachment irrespective of macular involvement.

d. Rubeosis iridis.

e. Severe persistent vitreous haemorrhage.

f. Macular oedema associated with tangential vitreoretinal traction.

A.

a. False. **b.** True (see above). **c.** True. **d.** False. **e.** True. **f.** True.

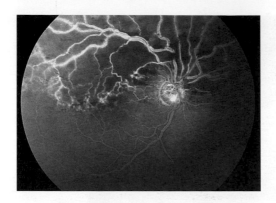

10   **Q. Branch retinal vein occlusion – true or false?**

a. Some cases may be asymptomatic.

b. Fluorescein angiography may show vascular staining and 'pruning' of vessels in ischaemic areas.

c. Intraretinal microvascular abnormalities characteristically develop across the horizontal raphe.

d. After 6 months 50% of eyes have a visual acuity of $^6/_{12}$ or better.

e. Cellophane maculopathy is the most common cause of persistent poor visual acuity.

f. Neovascularization should be treated without delay.

A.

a. True – only if a peripheral vein is involved. **b.** True (see above).
c. False – refers to collaterals. **d.** True. **e.** False. **f.** False.

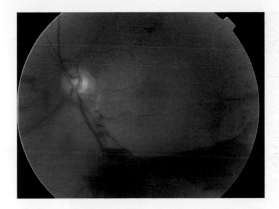

11 **Q. The following are causes of visual loss in retinal branch vein occlusion – true or false?**

a. Macular oedema.

b. Macular ischaemia.

c. Vitreous haemorrhage.

d. Neovascular glaucoma.

e. Macular lipid.

f. Choroidal neovascularization.

A.

a. True. **b.** True. **c.** True (see above). **d.** False. **e.** True. **f.** False.

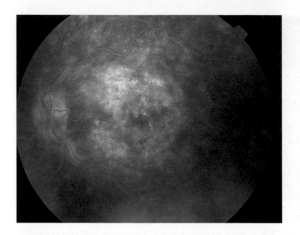

12 **Q. Non-ischaemic central retinal vein occlusion – true or false?**

a. It is more common than ischaemic central vein occlusion.

b. Afferent pupillary defect is absent.

c. Disc new vessels develop in 25% of cases within 6 months.

d. Eyes with chronic macular oedema (see above) and poor vision are treated with grid laser photocoagulation.

e. Most acute signs resolve within 6–12 months.

f. About one-third of cases convert to ischaemic central vein occlusion within 3 years.

A.

a. True – it accounts for 75% of cases. **b.** False – mild afferent defect may be present. **c.** False. **d.** False – laser is not beneficial. **e.** True. **f.** True.

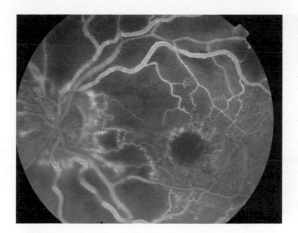

13 **Q. Ischaemic central retinal vein occlusion – true or false?**

a. Visual acuity is usually $^6/_{60}$ – CF.

b. Fluorescein angiography shows extensive retinal non-perfusion.

c. Development of disc collaterals may protect the eye from rubeosis iridis.

d. Angle new vessels may be present in the absence of rubeosis iridis.

e. Rubeosis iridis develops in about 50% of eyes, usually between 2 and 4 months.

f. All eyes with ischaemic central vein occlusion require urgent panretinal photocoagulation to prevent rubeosis iridis and neovascular glaucoma.

A.

a. False – CF or worse. **b.** True (see above). **c.** True. **d.** True. **e.** True.
f. False.

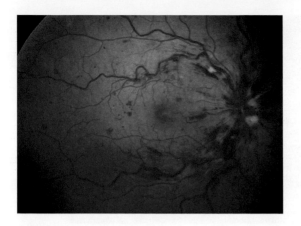

14   Q. Papillophlebitis – true or false?

a. Typically affects young patients with systemic vasculitis.

b. Disc oedema and peripapillary flame-shaped haemorrhages are the principal findings.

c. Visual acuity is relatively good.

d. Venous sheathing is characteristic.

e. Treatment involves systemic steroids.

f. Prognosis usually favourable.

A.

a. False – affects healthy patients. **b.** True (see above). **c.** True. **d.** False.
e. False. **f.** True.

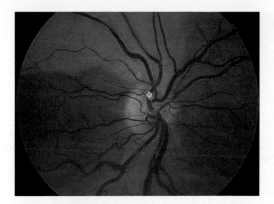

15   Q. Retinal artery occlusion – answer the following.

a. What is the most common underlying cause of central retinal artery occlusion?
b. What is the most common origin of retinal emboli?
c. What are Hollenhorst plaques?
d. What is the usual location of calcific emboli?
e. What is amaurosis fugax?
f. What is 'cattle-trucking'?

A.

a. Atherosclerosis-related thrombosis at the level of the lamina cribrosa.
b. Atheromatous plaque at the carotid bifurcation and less commonly from the aortic arch.   **c.** Cholesterol emboli which appear as intermittent showers of minute, bright, refractile, golden to yellow-orange crystals, often located at arteriolar bifurcations.   **d.** On or near the optic disc (see above).   **e.** Painless transient unilateral loss of vision usually caused by fibrin-platelet emboli.   **f.** Segmentation of the blood column.

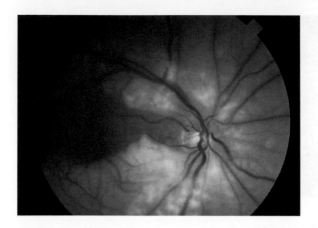

16 Q. Retinal artery occlusion – true or false?

a. Fluorescein angiography should be performed urgently.

b. Calcific emboli may cause permanent obstruction.

c. Giant cell arteritis is a common cause of branch occlusion.

d. Central artery occlusion may be associated with an amaurotic pupil.

e. In central retinal artery occlusion visual acuity may be normal.

f. Treatment of acute occlusion may involve anterior-chamber paracentesis.

A.

a. False. **b.** True. **c.** False. **d.** True. **e.** True – only if a cilioretinal artery is present (see above). **f.** True.

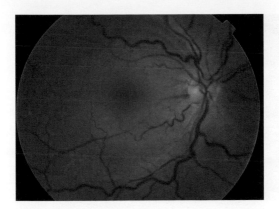

17 Q. Ocular ischaemic syndrome – true or false?

a. It is caused by ipsilateral atherosclerotic carotid stenosis of more than 90% that results in 50% reduction of ipsilateral perfusion pressure.

b. Majority of cases are bilateral.

c. Aqueous flare and cells may be present.

d. Rubeosis iridis is uncommon.

e. Venous dilatation and tortuosity may be present.

f. 5-year mortality is 40%.

A.

a. True. **b.** False – unilateral. **c.** True. **d.** False – common. **e.** True (see above). **f.** True.

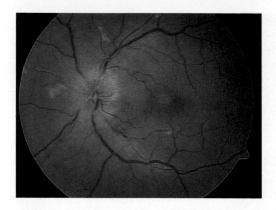

18 Q. Hypertensive disease – answer the following.

a. What is involutional sclerosis?

b. What is the most important sign of malignant hypertension?

c. What are the histological characteristics of arteriolosclerosis?

d. What are the signs of grade 2 arteriolosclerosis?

e. What is Gunn sign?

f. What are Elschnig spots?

A.

a. Age-related rigidity of retinal arterioles. **b.** Disc swelling (see above).
c. Intimal hyalinization, medial hypertrophy and endothelial hyperplasia.
d. Broadening of the arteriolar light reflex and deflection of veins at
arteriovenous crossings (Salus sign). **e.** Tapering of veins on both sides
of the crossings and right-angled deflection of veins. **f.** Small, black spots
surrounded by yellow halos which represent focal choroidal infarcts.

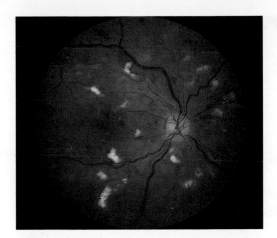

19 Q. The following may occur in hypertensive retinopathy – true or false?

a. Flame-shaped haemorrhages and cotton-wool spots.

b. Disc new vessels.

c. Cellophane maculopathy.

d. Macular star.

e. Venous tortuosity and dilatation.

f. Exudative retinal detachment.

A.

a. True (see above). **b.** False. **c.** False. **d.** True. **e.** False. **f.** True.

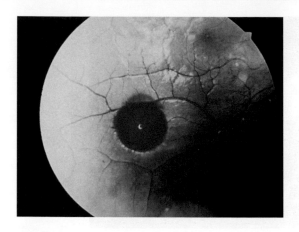

20 **Q. Sickle-cell retinopathy – true or false?**

a. Proliferative retinopathy is most severe in SC and SThal disease.
b. Most patients with proliferative retinopathy require argon laser photocoagulation.
c. Stage 2 proliferative disease is characterized by peripheral arteriovenous anastomoses of dilated pre-existent capillary channels.
d. Black sunbursts are patches of peripheral RPE hyperplasia.
e. Salmon patches are haemorrhages at the macula.
f. Angioid streaks are common in non-proliferative retinopathy.

A.

a. True. **b.** False. **c.** True. **d.** True. **e.** False – equator (see above).
f. False.

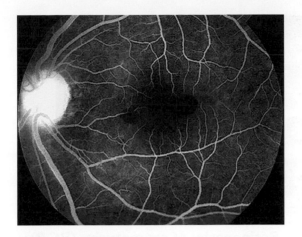

21 **Q. The following may cause visual loss in sickle-cell retinopathy – true or false?**

a. Tractional retinal detachment.

b. Macular ischaemia.

c. Cystoid macular oedema.

d. Vitreous haemorrhage.

e. Anterior ischaemic optic neuropathy.

f. Macular lipid.

A.

a. True. **b.** True (see above). **c.** False. **d.** True. **e.** False. **f.** False.

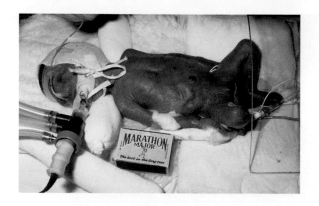

22 Q. Retinopathy of prematurity (ROP) – answer the following.

a. What is ROP?

b. When does retinal vascularization normally commence?

c. When does vascularization of the temporal periphery become complete?

d. What is the incidence of spontaneous regression?

e. Which babies require screening?

f. What is threshold disease?

A.

a. A proliferative retinopathy affecting premature infants of very low birth weight, who have often been exposed to high oxygen concentrations.

b. Fourth month of gestation. **c.** One month after delivery. **d.** About 80% of cases regress spontaneously. **e.** Screening is required of babies born at or before 31 weeks' gestational age, or weighing 1500 g or less (see above). **f.** 5 contiguous clock hours or 8 cumulative clock hours of extraretinal neovascularization (stage 3 disease) in zone 1 or zone 2, associated with plus disease.

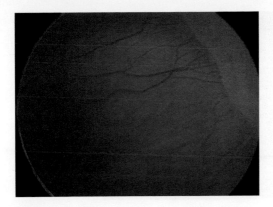

23   Q. ROP – true or false?

a. Zone 1 is bounded by an imaginary circle the radius of which is twice the distance from the disc to the macula.

b. Stage 2 is characterized by a ridge that arises in the region of the demarcation line.

c. Stage 4a active disease is characterized by a partial retinal detachment that involves the fovea.

d. Untreated rush disease usually progresses to retinal detachment.

e. Cryotherapy induces less myopia than laser photocoagulation.

f. About 20% of infants with active ROP develop cicatricial complications.

A.

a. True. **b.** True (see above). **c.** False — fovea is spared. **d.** True. **e.** False — reverse applies. **f.** True.

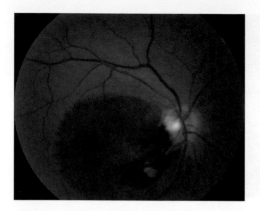

24   Q. Retinal artery macroaneurysm – true or false?

a. Typically occurs in elderly diabetic men.

b. It is usually unilateral.

c. Multiple macroaneurysms in the same eye are common.

d. May cause sudden visual loss.

e. Spontaneous involution is common.

f. Treatment involves cryotherapy.

A.

a. False – elderly hypertensive females. **b.** True. **c.** False. **d.** True
(see above). **e.** True. **f.** False – laser photocoagulation.

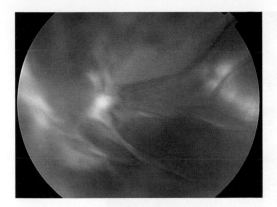

25   Q. Coats disease – true or false?

a. Majority of patients are males.

b. Average age at presentation is 5 years.

c. May be associated with atypical pigmentary retinopathy.

d. All cases are progressive and require treatment.

e. The prognosis is poor in older patients.

f. May give rise to retinal detachment.

A.

a. True. **b.** True. **c.** True. **d.** False. **e.** False – in patients under the age of 3 years. **f.** True (see above).

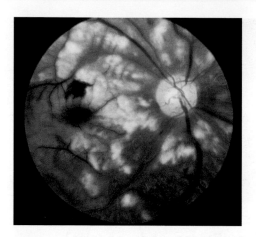

26   Q. Miscellaneous retinal vascular disorders – answer the following.

a. At what age and in which way does Eales disease present?

b. What is the treatment of radiation papillopathy?

c. What is the most common cause of Purtscher retinopathy?

d. What are the fundus changes in Purtscher retinopathy?

e. What are the signs of Valsalva retinopathy?

f. What is lipaemia retinalis?

A.

a. In the third to fifth decades with vitreous haemorrhage. **b.** Systemic steroids. **c.** Severe trauma, especially to the head and chest compressive injury. **d.** Multiple, unilateral or bilateral, superficial, white retinal patches, resembling large cotton-wool spots (see above). **e.** Unilateral or bilateral premacular haemorrhages. **f.** Creamy white retinal blood vessels in patients with hypertriglyceridaemia.

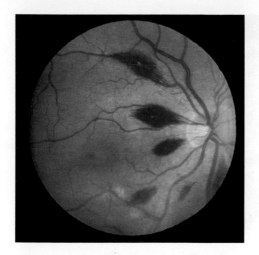

27 **Q. Roth spots occur in the following – true or false?**

a. Bacterial endocarditis.

b. Lupus retinopathy.

c. Radiation retinopathy.

d. Behçet disease.

e. Leukaemia.

f. HIV retinopathy.

A.

a. True. b. False. c. False. d. False. e. True (see above). f. True.

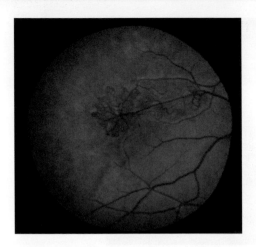

28 **Q. The following are causes of peripheral retinal neovascularization – true or false?**

a. Sarcoidosis.

b. Chronic myeloid leukaemia.

c. Sickle-cell retinopathy.

d. Harada disease.

e. Eales disease.

f. Hyperviscosity.

A.

a. True. **b.** True. **c.** True (see above). **d.** False. **e.** True. **f.** False.

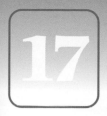
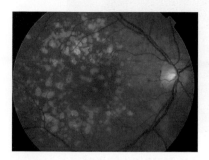

1 **Q. Age-related macular degeneration (ARMD) – answer the following.**

a. What percentage of patients aged over 85 years are blind from ARMD?

b. What are drusen (see above)?

c. What is the diameter of soft drusen?

d. What is the pathogenesis of atrophic (dry) ARMD?

e. What is the pathogenesis of neovascular (wet) ARMD?

f. What were the compounds used in the AREDS study?

A.

a. 18%. **b.** Discrete deposits of the abnormal material located between the basal lamina of the retinal pigment epithelium (RPE) and the inner collagenous layer of Bruch membrane. **c.** One vein width or more.

d. Slowly progressive atrophy of the photoreceptors, RPE and choriocapillaris.

e. Choroidal neovascularization (CNV) originating from the choriocapillaris, which grows through defects in Bruch membrane. **f.** 500 mg of vitamin C, 400 IU of vitamin E, 15 mg of beta carotene, 80 mg of zinc as zinc oxide and 2 mg of copper as cupric acid to prevent potential anaemia.

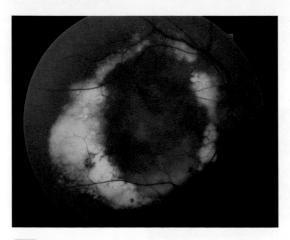

2   Q. Wet ARMD – true or false?

a. It is more common than dry.

b. Fluorescein angiography of classic CNV shows 'lacy' pattern in the early frames.

c. Most subfoveal CNV are classic.

d. Occult CNV is a poorly defined with less precise features on the early frames but gives rise to late, diffuse or multifocal leakage

e. It may give rise to extensive subretinal lipid exudation.

f. Retinal angiomatous proliferation is an uncommon manifestation of wet ARMD in which the neovascular process originates from the retinal vasculature as opposed to the choriocapillaris.

A.

a. False. **b.** True. **c.** False. **d.** True. **e.** True (see above). **f.** True.

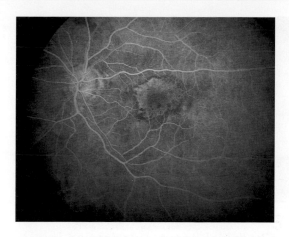

3 Q. Treatment of wet ARMD – true or false?

a. Photodynamic therapy (PDT) may be used for classic subfoveal CNV (see above).

b. In PDT the spot size is 500 μm larger than the diameter of CNV.

c. Recurrence rate following PDT within 12 weeks is 94%.

d. Macular translocation is more appropriate than subretinal surgery.

e. Anti-VEGF agents may be used in combination with PDT.

f. Anecortave acetate is given by anterior sub-Tenon injection.

A.

a. True. **b.** False – 1000 μm larger. **c.** True. **d.** True. **e.** True. **f.** False – posterior sub-Tenon injection.

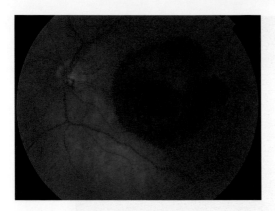

4   **Q. Choroidal neovascularization in ARMD may result in the following – true or false?**

a. Haemorrhagic RPE detachment.

b. Vitreous haemorrhage.

c. Subretinal scarring.

d. Exudative retinal detachment.

e. Vitreomacular traction.

f. Macular epiretinal membrane formation.

A.

a. True (see above). **b.** True. **c.** True. **d.** True. **e.** False. **f.** False.

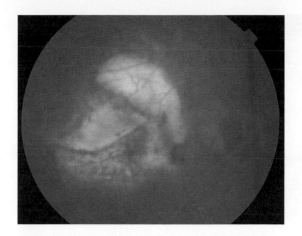

5 Q. Detachment of the RPE may be associated with the following – true or false?

a. Subsequent geographic atrophy.

b. Detachment of the sensory retina.

c. Tear of the RPE.

d. Cystoid macular oedema.

e. Classic CNV.

f. Spontaneous resolution.

A.

a. True. **b.** True. **c.** True (see above). **d.** False. **e.** False – occult CNV.
f. True.

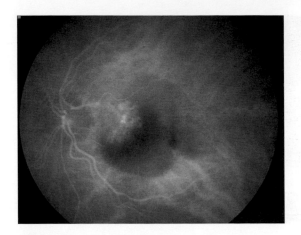

6   **Q. Polypoidal choroidal vasculopathy – true or false?**

a. Presentation is in old age.

b. Involvement is often bilateral and symmetrical in severity.

c. The two main types are exudative and haemorrhagic.

d. Most lesions are peripapillary.

e. Fluorescein angiography is superior to indocyanine angiography in delineating the polyps.

f. The prognosis is good in 50% of cases with eventual spontaneous resolution.

A.

a. True. **b.** False – asymmetrical. **c.** True. **d.** False – at the macula.
e. False – indocyanine green angiography is required to make the diagnosis (see above). **f.** True.

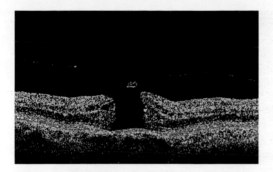

7 **Q. Age-related (idiopathic) macular hole – true or false?**

a. Involvement of the fellow eye at 5 years is about 25%.

b. Stage 3 is characterized by a full-thickness defect greater than 400 μm in diameter with an attached posterior hyaloid face, with or without an overlying pseudo-operculum.

c. Retinal detachment at the macula occurs in 5% after 10 years.

d. Fluorescein angiography is more accurate in the diagnosis of a stage 4 macular hole than optical coherence tomography.

e. Some holes may close spontaneously.

f. Indications for surgery are stage 2 and above holes with a visual acuity worse than ⁶/₉.

A.

a. False – 10%. **b.** True (see above). **c.** False. **d.** False. **e.** True. **f.** True.

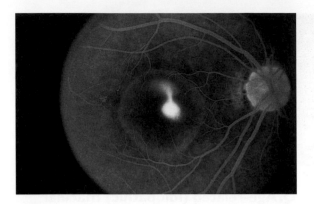

8   Q. Central serous retinopathy – true or false?

a. Typically affects young women with type A personality.

b. Micropsia is more common than macropsia.

c. Optical coherence tomography is essential for diagnosis.

d. In most cases, the subretinal fluid absorbs spontaneously within 3–6 months and visual acuity returns to normal or near-normal.

e. On fluorescein angiography the 'smoke-stack' appearance (see above) is less common than the 'ink-blot'.

f. Congenital optic disc pit should be considered in the differential diagnosis.

A.

a. False – young men with type A personality. **b.** True. **c.** False. **d.** True.

e. False – reverse applies. **f.** True.

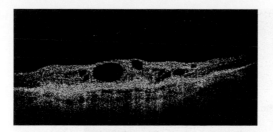

9   Q. Cystoid macular oedema – true or false?

a. Most cases are idiopathic.

b. The diagnosis cannot usually be made on slit-lamp examination alone.

c. A 'flower petal' pattern of hyperfluorescence is characteristic on fluorescein angiography.

d. Systemic carbonic anhydrase inhibitors may be beneficial in selected cases.

e. Optical coherence topography (see above) is more useful than fluorescein angiography in assessing progression.

f. Pars plana vitrectomy may be useful for cases refractory to medical therapy even in eyes without apparent vitreous disturbance.

A.

a. False. **b.** False. **c.** True. **d.** True. **e.** True. **f.** True.

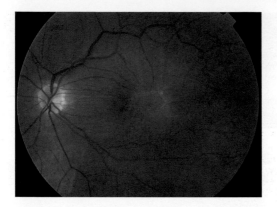

10   Q. Macular epiretinal membranes – true or false?

a. Idiopathic membranes typically affect elderly individuals and are bilateral in 10% of cases.

b. They typically occur in myopic eyes.

c. Cellophane maculopathy is less serious than macular pucker.

d. Vascular distortion at the macula is the key to diagnosis.

e. Secondary membranes may develop following glaucoma filtration surgery.

f. Surgical removal usually improves distortion but rarely improves visual acuity.

A.

a. True. **b.** False. **c.** True. **d.** True (see above). **e.** False. **f.** False – visual acuity improves in 50% of cases.

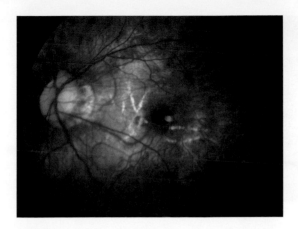

11 Q. Degenerative myopia – true or false?

a. It is defined as an eye with a refractive error >-6D and an axial length of the globe >26 mm.

b. Retinal detachment is the most common cause of visual loss.

c. Lacquer cracks are innocuous.

d. Fuchs spot is a raised, circular, pigmented lesion that may develops after a macular haemorrhage has absorbed.

e. It is associated with an increased prevalence of primary open-angle glaucoma.

f. Macular holes in myopic eyes never give rise to retinal detachment.

A.

a. True. **b.** False – maculopathy. **c.** False – predispose to CNV (see above). **d.** True. **e.** True. **f.** False.

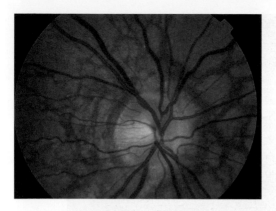

12 Q. Angioid streaks – answer the following.

a. What are angioid streaks (see above)?

b. What is 'peau d'orange?

c. What are the findings on fluorescein angiography?

d. What congenital optic nerve condition may be seen in eyes with angioid streaks?

e. What is the most common cause of visual loss?

f. What is Grönblad–Strandberg syndrome?

A.

a. Crack-like dehiscences in the thickened, calcified and abnormally brittle collagenous and elastic portions of Bruch membrane. **b.** Mottled pigmentation at the posterior pole more marked temporally.

c. Hyperfluorescence caused by RPE window defects over the streaks.

d. Optic disc drusen. **e.** CNV. **f.** Association of angioid streaks with pseudoxanthoma elasticum.

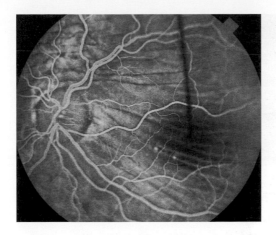

13 Q. Miscellaneous maculopathies – true or false?

a. Idiopathic choroidal folds usually occur in hypermetropic eyes.

b. Longstanding choroidal folds may be associated with CNV.

c. Fluorescein angiography in choroidal folds shows hypofluorescence corresponds to the crests and hyperfluorescence corresponding to the troughs (see above).

d. Glaucoma filtration surgery with adjunctive antimetabolites is the most common cause of hypotony maculopathy.

e. Pars plana vitrectomy for vitreomacular traction syndrome is seldom beneficial.

f. Severe bilateral solar maculopathy usually responds to a short course of low-dose systemic steroids.

A.

a. True. **b.** False. **c.** False – reverse applies **d.** True. **e.** False. **f.** False.

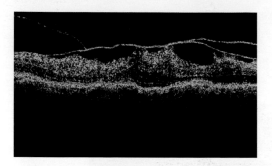

14   **Q. The following may be associated with cystoid macular oedema – true or false?**

a. Vitreoretinal traction syndrome.

b. Intermediate uveitis.

c. Retinitis pigmentosa.

d. Branch retinal vein occlusion.

e. Secondary intraocular lens implantation.

f. YAG laser capsulotomy.

A.

a. True (see above).   **b.** True.   **c.** True.   **d.** True.   **e.** True.   **f.** True.

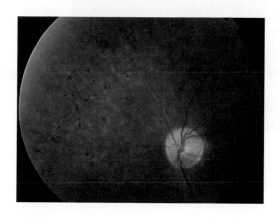

1 **Q. Retinitis pigmentosa (RP) – answer the following.**

a. What is RP?
b. What mode of inheritance has the best prognosis?
c. What mode of inheritance has the worst prognosis?
d. What is the classic triad of RP?
e. What is the typical visual field defect?
f. What does the ERG show in early cases?

A.

a. RP defines a clinically and genetically diverse group of diffuse retinal dystrophies initially predominantly affecting the rod photoreceptor cells with subsequent degeneration of cones. **b.** AD. **c.** X-linked. **d.** Arteriolar attenuation, bone spicule pigmentation and waxy disc pallor (see above). **e.** Annular mid-peripheral scotoma. **f.** Reduced scotopic rod and combined responses.

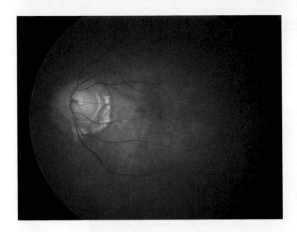

2   Q. RP – true or false?

a. Female carriers of X-linked RP have normal fundi.

b. Associated cystoid macular oedema in RP may respond to systemic steroids.

c. Associated systemic conditions are usually AR.

d. Rarely pigmentary changes may be sparse or absent.

e. Colour vision is normal.

f. Electro-oculography is normal.

A.

a. False – may have a golden-metallic reflex at the macula. **b.** False – may respond to oral acetazolamide. **c.** True. **d.** True (see above). **e.** True.
f. False – the light rise is absent.

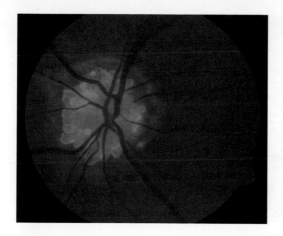

3   Q. The following may occur in RP – true or false?

a. Open-angle glaucoma.

b. Optic disc drusen.

c. Chronic anterior uveitis.

d. Myopia.

e. Cellophane maculopathy.

f. Coats-like vasculopathy.

A.

a. True. **b.** True (see above). **c.** False. **d.** True. **e.** True. **f.** True.

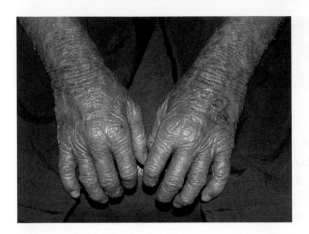

4   **Q. Match the systemic association of RP (a–f) with the appropriate feature (i–vi).**

a. Bassen–Kornzweig syndrome.

b. Refsum disease.

c. Usher syndrome.

d. Kearns–Sayre syndrome.

e. Bardet–Biedl syndrome.

f. Friedreich ataxia.

i. Deafness.

ii. Heart block.

iii. Acanthocytosis.

iv. Ichthyosis (see above).

v. Deformed feet.

vi. Polydactyly.

A.

a. & **iii**;   **b.** & **iv**;   **c.** & **i**;   **d.** & **ii**;   **e.** & **vi**;   **f.** & **v**.

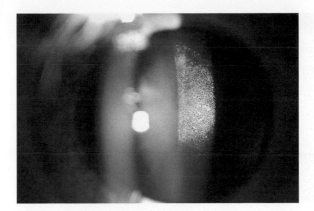

5 **Q. Cone dystrophy – true or false?**

a. The rod system remains unaffected.

b. Most cases are sporadic.

c. Bull's eye maculopathy is universal.

d. Photopic ERG is subnormal or non-recordable.

e. Colour vision is impaired early.

f. Posterior subcapsular cataracts (see above) develop by the fifth decade.

A.

a. False. **b.** True. **c.** False. **d.** True. **e.** True. **f.** False.

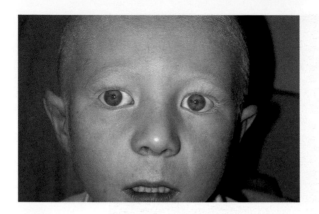

6   Q. Albinism – true or false?

a. Tyrosinase-positive oculocutaneous albinos have a 'pink eyed' appearance (see above).

b. Albinos have an increased risk of cutaneous melanoma.

c. Most patients with tyrosinase-negative oculocutaneous albinism develop open-angle glaucoma by the fourth decade of life.

d. In tyrosinase-positive oculocutaneous albinism the optic chiasm has fewer uncrossed nerve fibres than normal, so that the majority of fibres from each eye cross to the contralateral hemisphere.

e. Poor vision in ocular albinism is caused by foveal hypoplasia.

f. Inheritance of ocular albinism is usually X-linked.

A.

a. False – tyrosinase negative. **b.** False – cutaneous basal cell and squamous-cell carcinoma. **c.** False. **d.** False – tyrosinase-negative.
e. False – applies to oculocutaneous albinism. **f.** True.

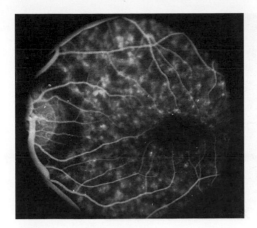

7   Q. Stargardt disease and fundus flavimaculatus – true or false?

a. They are regarded as variants of the same disease despite presenting at different times and carrying different prognoses.

b. Prognosis is better in the former than the latter.

c. Inheritance of both is AR.

d. Fluorescein angiography shows a 'dark choroid' in the latter but not the former.

e. Fundus autofluorescence may be seen in the latter but not the former.

f. Both conditions show a subnormal photopic and scotopic ERG.

A.

a. True. **b.** False – reverse applies. **c.** True. **d.** False – both show a 'dark choroid' (see above). **e.** True. **f.** False – photopic ERG is normal to subnormal and scotopic is normal.

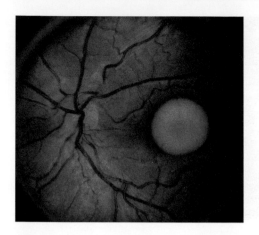

8   **Q. Juvenile Best macular dystrophy –
true or false?**

a. Inheritance is AD.

b. ERG may be subnormal in asymptomatic patients with normal fundi.

c. Stage 1 is characterized by a round egg-yolk ('sunny side up') macular lesion (see above).

d. Visual acuity begins to deteriorate in stage 4.

e. Involvement may be asymmetrical.

f. Choroidal neovascularization may occasionally cause severe visual loss.

A.

a. True. **b.** False – applies to the EOG. **c.** False – applies to stage 2.
d. True. **e.** True. **f.** True.

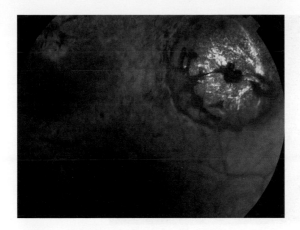

9 **Q. Leber congenital amaurosis – true or false?**

a. Inheritance is X-linked or AD.

b. Pupillary light reflexes may be absent.

c. Fundi may be normal despite very poor vision.

d. ERG is normal in early cases.

e. Macular coloboma-like atrophy may be present.

f. Enophthalmos may be present.

A.

a. False – AR. **b.** True. **c.** True. **d.** False. **e.** True (see above). **f.** True – due to constant eye rubbing (oculodigital syndrome).

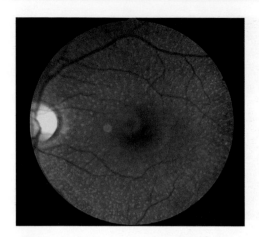

10 **Q. Match the following description (a–f) with the appropriate condition (i–vi).**

a. Bilateral exudative maculopathy in the fifth decade.
b. Confluent drusen-like macular deposits.

c. Fluorescein angiography shows central hypofluorescence surrounded by a small irregular hyperfluorescent ring.
d. Yellow pigment at the fovea arranged in a triradiate pattern.
e. Scattered perimacular and peripheral flecks, and anterior lenticonus.
f. Congenital stationary night-blindness.

i. North Carolina macular dystrophy.
ii. Sorsby pseudo-inflammatory macular dystrophy.
iii. Adult-onset foveomacular vitelliform dystrophy.
iv. Butterfly-shaped macular dystrophy.
v. Fundus albipunctatus.
vi. Alport syndrome.

A.

a. & **ii**; **b.** & **i**; **c.** & **iii**; **d.** & **iv**; **e.** & **vi**; **f.** & **v** (see above).

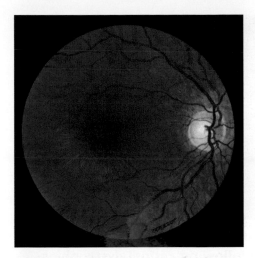

11 Q. Congenital retinoschisis – answer the following.

a. What is the basic defect?

b. How does it differ from acquired retinoschisis?

c. What is the appearance of maculopathy?

d. What percentage of patients has peripheral schisis?

e. What are ERG findings in peripheral schisis?

f. What are 'vitreous veils'?

A.

a. In Müller cells, causing splitting of the retinal nerve fibre layer from the rest of the sensory retina. **b.** In acquired retinoschisis the splitting occurs at the outer plexiform layer. **c.** Cystoid spaces with a 'bicycle-wheel' pattern of radial striae (see above). **d.** 50%. **e.** Decrease in amplitude of the b-wave as compared with the a-wave on scotopic and photopic testing. **f.** Floating retinal blood vessels following disintegration of the schisis.

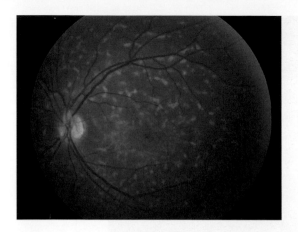

12 Q. The following retinal dystrophies carry a favourable visual prognosis – true or false?

a. Fundus albipunctatus.

b. Fundus flavimaculatus (see above).

c. Fundus pulverulentus.

d. Retinitis punctata albescens.

e. Butterfly dystrophy.

f. Adult-onset foveomacular vitelliform dystrophy.

A.

a. True. **b.** False. **c.** True. **d.** False. **e.** True. **f.** True.

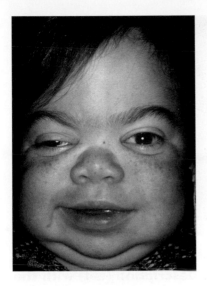

13 **Q. The following may be associated with bull's eye maculopathy – true or false?**

a. Batten disease.

b. Usher syndrome.

c. Tay–Sachs disease.

d. Hurler syndrome (see above).

e. Bardet–Biedl syndrome.

f. Hallervorden–Spatz disease.

A.

a. True. b. False. c. False. d. False. e. True. f. True.

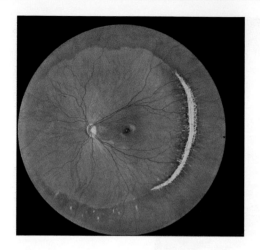

14   Q. Match the description (a–f) with the appropriate condition (i–vi).

a. Radial lattice-like degeneration associated with RPE hyperplasia, vascular sheathing and sclerosis.

i. Wagner syndrome.

b. Vascular straightening and temporal dragging of the macula and disc.

ii. Favre–Goldmann disease.

c. Retinoschisis and pigmentary retinopathy.

iii. Familial exudative vitreoretinopathy.

d. X-linked recessive inheritance.

iv. Gyrate atrophy

e. Elevated serum ornithine.

v. Stickler syndrome.

f. Low myopia and empty vitreous.

vi. Choroideremia.

A.

a. & **v**; **b.** & **iii** (see above); **c.** & **ii**; **d.** & **vi**; **e.** & **iv**; **f.** & **i**.

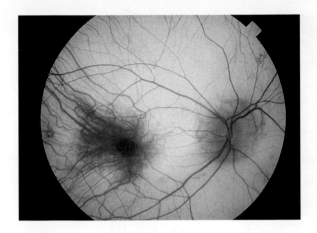

15 Q. Choroidal dystrophies – true or false?

a. Female carriers of choroideremia have normal ERG.

b. Choroideremia starts in the extreme fundus periphery.

c. Female carriers of choroideremia have subnormal EOG.

d. In choroideremia the fovea is spared until late and the optic disc and retinal vasculature remain relatively normal.

e. Cystoid macular oedema may occur in gyrate atrophy.

f. Most patients with central areolar choroidal dystrophy become legally blind by middle age.

A.

a. True. **b.** False – midperiphery. **c.** False. **d.** True (see above). **e.** True. **f.** False – old age.

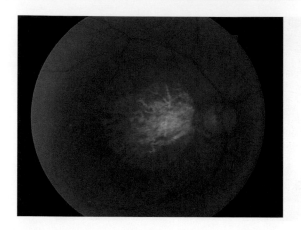

16 Q. The following have a normal ERG – true or false?

a. Central areolar choroidal dystrophy (see above).

b. Butterfly-shaped macular dystrophy.

c. Dominant macular oedema.

d. North Carolina macular dystrophy.

e. Familial drusen.

f. Juvenile Best macular dystrophy.

A.

a. True. **b.** True. **c.** True. **d.** True. **e.** True. **f.** True.

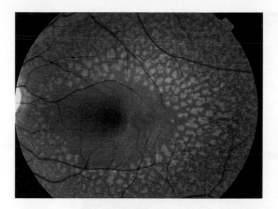

17 **Q. The following are autosomal recessive – true or false?**

a. Stickler syndrome.

b. Fundus flavimaculatus.

c. Congenital retinoschisis.

d. Sorsby pseudo-inflammatory macular dystrophy.

e. Leber congenital amaurosis.

f. Benign familial flecked retina (see above).

A.

a. False – AD. **b.** True. **c.** False – X-linked. **d.** False – AD. **e.** True.
f. True.

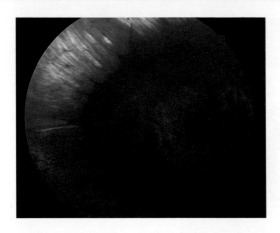

18 **Q. Match the diet (a–d) with the appropriate condition (i–iv).**

a. Vitamin B6.   **i.** Refsum disease.
b. Vitamin A.   **ii.** RP.
c. Vitamin E.   **iii.** Gyrate atrophy (see above).
d. Phytanic acid-free.   **iv.** Bassen-Kornzweig syndrome.

A.
a. & **iii**; **b.** & **ii**; **c.** & **iv**; **d.** & **i**.

CHAPTER 19 **Retinal detachment**

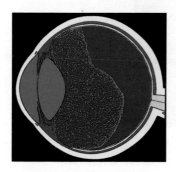

1 Q. Define the following conditions.

a. Retinal detachment (RD).
b. Rhegmatogenous RD.
c. Tractional RD.
d. Retinal break.
e. Dynamic vitreoretinal traction.
f. Posterior vitreous detachment.

A.

a. Separation of the neurosensory retina from the retinal pigment epithelium (RPE). **b.** RD caused by a full-thickness defect in the sensory retina. **c.** RD in which the sensory retina is pulled away from the RPE by contracting vitreoretinal membranes in the absence of a retinal break. **d.** Full-thickness defect in the sensory retina. **e.** Dynamic vitreoretinal traction is induced by eye movements and exerts a centripetal force towards the vitreous cavity. **f.** Separation of the cortical vitreous from the internal limiting membrane of the sensory retina posterior to the vitreous base (see above).

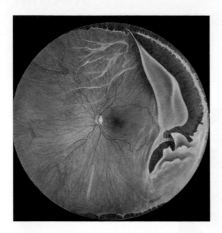

2   Q. Retinal breaks – true or false?

a. Tears are caused by static vitreoretinal traction.

b. Tears have a predilection for the upper temporal fundus.

c. Holes are usually found inferiorly.

d. Macular breaks are usually holes.

e. Dialyses are circumferential tears along the ora serrata with the vitreous gel attached to their posterior margins.

f. Giant tears involve more than 45° of the fundus.

A.

a. False – dynamic vitreoretinal traction. **b.** True. **c.** False. **d.** True.

e. True. **f.** False – involve at least 90° (see above).

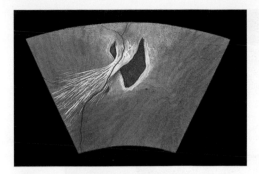

3 **Q. Pathogenesis of rhegmatogenous RD – true or false?**

a. Retinal breaks responsible for RD are caused by interplay between dynamic vitreoretinal traction and an underlying weakness in the peripheral retina referred to as predisposing degeneration.

b. RD is eventually bilateral in 25% of patients.

c. Retinal tears (see above) develop in 10–15% of eyes with acute posterior vitreous detachment.

d. RD never occurs in the absence of acute posterior vitreous detachment.

e. About 60% of all breaks develop in areas of the peripheral retina that shows specific changes.

f. Most breaks do not result in RD.

A.

a. True. **b.** False – eventually bilateral in 10% of cases. **c.** True. **d.** False. **e.** True. **f.** True.

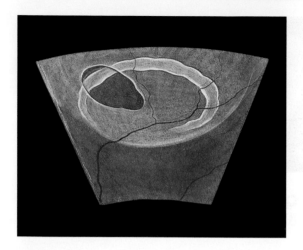

4 Q. Predisposing peripheral degenerations – true or false?

a. Lattice degeneration typically affects elderly patients.

b. Holes within lattice lesions are common and usually innocuous.

c. Snailtrack degeneration is frequently associated with U-shaped tears.

d. Degenerative retinoschisis rarely causes RD.

e. Breaks in the inner layer of retinoschisis are usually large and have rolled edges.

f. 'White-without-pressure' may be associated with giant tear formation.

A.

a. False. **b.** True. **c.** False – round holes. **d.** True. **e.** False – outer layer breaks (see above). **f.** True.

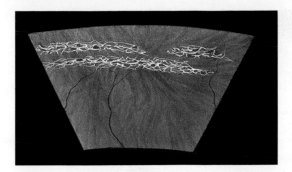

5 Q. Significance of myopia in RD – true or false?

a. About 20% of the population are myopic.

b. Over 40% of all RD occur in myopic eyes.

c. There is no correlation between the degree of myopia and the risk of RD.

d. Lattice degeneration (see above) is more common in myopic eyes.

e. Macular holes in myopic eyes may give rise to RD.

f. Diffuse chorioretinal atrophy may give rise to small round holes in highly myopic eyes.

A.

a. False – 10%. b. True. c. False – high myopia carries a greater risk.
d. True. e. True. f. True.

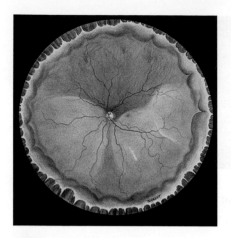

6   **Q. The following may cause exudative RD – true or false?**

a. Melanoma of the choroid.

b. Blunt ocular trauma.

c. Eclampsia.

d. Posterior scleritis.

e. Uveal effusion syndrome.

f. Proliferative diabetic retinopathy.

A.

a. True. **b.** False. **c.** True. **d.** True. **e.** True (see above). **f.** False – tractional RD.

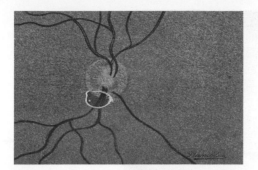

7 Q. Clinical features of rhegmatogenous RD – answer the following.

a. What are the classic premonitory symptoms of acute posterior vitreous detachment?

b. What is a Weiss ring?

c. What is 'tobacco dust'?

d. What is the significance of secondary intraretinal cysts?

e. What are 'high water marks'?

f. What are the signs of grade 2 proliferative vitreoretinopathy?

A.

a. Flashing lights (photopsia) and vitreous floaters. **b.** Solitary floater consisting of the detached annular attachment of vitreous to the margin of the optic disc (see above). **c.** RPE cells and macrophages in the retrolental space. **d.** They occur in long-standing RD. **e.** Demarcation lines caused by proliferation of RPE cells at the junction of flat and detached retina. **f.** Wrinkling of the inner retinal surface, tortuosity of blood vessels, retinal stiffness, decreased mobility of vitreous gel and rolled edges of retinal breaks.

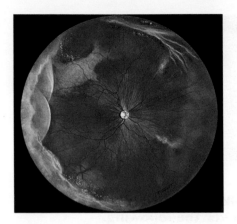

8   **Q. Differential diagnosis of RD – true or false?**

a. Tractional RD shows the phenomenon of 'shifting fluid'.
b. Subretinal fluid is deeper in tractional than in rhegmatogenous RD.
c. 'Leopard spots' consisting of scattered areas of subretinal clumping may be seen after an exudative RD has flattened.
d. Degenerative retinoschisis rarely extends beyond the equator.
e. Holes in the inner layer of degenerative retinoschisis are common.
f. Uveal effusion syndrome is characterized by exudative retinal and choroidal detachment.

A.

a. False – applies to exudative RD. **b.** False – reverse applies. **c.** True.
d. True (see above). **e.** True. **f.** True.

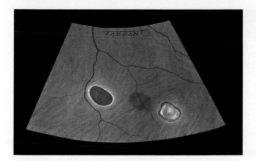

9 **Q. Prophylaxis of RD – list these lesions in decreasing risk of progression to RD.**

a. Large symptomatic U-tear in the upper temporal quadrant.

b. Two small asymptomatic holes near the inferior ora serrata.

c. Superior giant tear in a highly myopic eye.

d. U-tear at 6 o'clock with a detached operculum (see above).

e. Degenerative retinoschisis with breaks in both layers.

f. Large asymptomatic U-tear in the inferior nasal quadrant.

A.

c., a., f., d., e. and **b.**

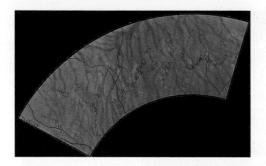

10   **Q. The following peripheral retinal degenerations are innocuous – true or false?**

a. Microcystoid.

b. Pavingstone.

c. Honeycomb (see above).

d. Snowflake.

e. Snailtrack.

f. Oral pigmentary.

A.

a. True. **b.** True. **c.** True. **d.** True. **e.** False. **f.** True.

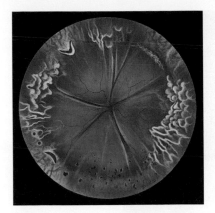

11 Q. Surgery for rhegmatogenous RD – answer the following.

a. What is pneumatic retinopexy?

b. What does scleral buckling involve?

c. From which material are explants made?

d. What is the most serious operative complication of drainage of subretinal fluid?

e. What are the two most common causes of early failure?

f. What is the most common cause of late failure?

A.

a. An intravitreal expanding gas bubble is used to seal a retinal break and reattach the retina without scleral buckling. **b.** Material sutured onto the sclera (explant) creates an inward indentation (buckle). **c.** Silicone, which may be soft or hard. **d.** Retinal incarceration. **e.** Missed retinal break or buckle failure. **f.** Proliferative vitreoretinopathy (see above).

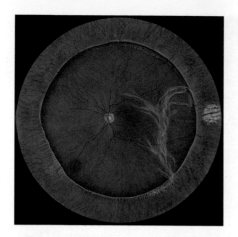

12 Q. Match the condition (a–f) with the appropriate operation (i–vi).

a. Small symptomatic U-tear.

b. U-tear associated with shallow subretinal fluid.

c. Giant tear and retinal detachment.

d. Traumatic dialysis and retinal detachment.

e. RD with breaks in three quadrants.

f. Severe proliferative vitreoretinopathy.

i. Pars plana vitrectomy, membrane dissection and extended intraocular tamponade.

ii. Laser or cryotherapy.

iii. Encircling buckle (see above).

iv. Circumferential buckle.

v. Cryotherapy and radial buckle.

vi. Pars plana vitrectomy, injection of heavy liquid and endolaser.

A.

a. & **ii**; **b.** & **v**; **c.** & **vi**; **d.** & **iv**; **e.** & **iii**; **f.** & **i**.

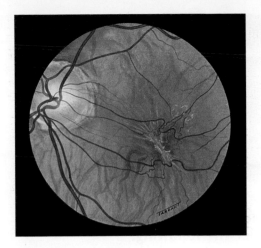

13 Q. Complications of scleral buckling –
true or false?

a. Diplopia.

b. Anterior segment ischaemia.

c. Glaucoma.

d. Intermediate uveitis.

e. Orbital cellulitis.

f. Macular pucker.

A.

a. True. b. True. c. True. d. False. e. True. f. True (see above).

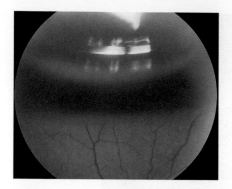

14   Q. Principles of pars plana vitrectomy – answer the following.

a. What is the diameter of the shafts of most instruments?

b. What is the purpose of intraocular gas injection (see above)?

c. What are the properties of heavy liquids?

d. For how many days does sulphahexafluoride remain in the eye?

e. What is delamination?

f. What is segmentation?

A.

a. 0.9 mm (20-guage). **b.** To produce internal tamponade of retinal breaks during the postoperative period. **c.** They have a high specific gravity and thus remain in a dependent position when injected into the vitreous cavity. **d.** 10–14 days. **e.** Horizontal cutting of the individual vascular pegs connecting the membranes to the surface of the retina. **f.** Vertical cutting of epiretinal membranes into small segments.

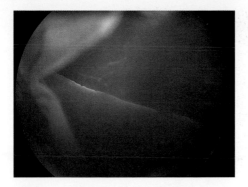

15 **Q. Indications for pars plana vitrectomy – true or false?**

a. Tractional RD threatening the macula.

b. Failed scleral buckling.

c. Severe proliferative vitreoretinopathy.

d. RD due to large posterior tears (see above).

e. Combined tractional-rhegmatogenous RD.

f. Recent rhegmatogenous RD and dense vitreous haemorrhage.

A.

a. True. **b.** False. **c.** True. **d.** True. **e.** True. **f.** True.

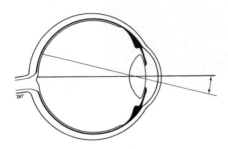

1   Q. Define the following.

a. Orthophoria.
b. Heterophoria (phoria).
c. Heterotropia (tropia).
d. Visual axis (line of vision).
e. Anatomical axis.
f. Angle kappa.

A.

a. Perfect ocular alignment in the absence of any stimulus for fusion.
b. Tendency of the eyes to deviate when fusion is blocked (latent squint).
c. Manifest deviation in which the visual axes do not intersect at the point of fixation. **d.** Line passing from the fovea, through the nodal point of the eye to the point of fixation (object of regard). **e.** Line passing from the posterior pole through the centre of the cornea. **f.** Angle subtended by the visual and anatomical axes (see above).

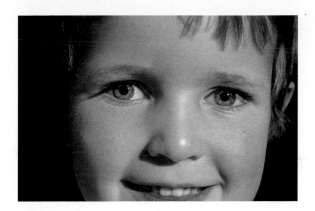

2 Q. True or false?

a. Angle kappa is positive when the fovea is nasal to the centre of the posterior pole resulting in a temporal displacement of the corneal reflex.

b. Large angle kappa may give the appearance of a squint when none is present (pseudosquint).

c. Large angle kappa may result in pseudo-esotropia following displacement of the macula in retinopathy of prematurity.

d. Listing plane is an imaginary sagittal plane passing through the centre of rotation of the globe.

e. The globe rotates left and right on the vertical Z axis of Fick.

f. The globe rotates up and down on the horizontal X axis of Fick.

A.

a. False – opposite applies. **b.** True. **c.** False – pseudo-exotropia (see above). **d.** False – coronal plane. **e.** True. **f.** True.

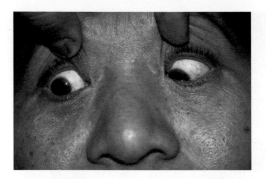

3 **Q. The following muscles are involved in dextrodepression – true or false?**

a. Right inferior rectus and left superior oblique.

b. Right superior rectus and left inferior oblique.

c. Right inferior rectus and left inferior oblique.

d. Right superior oblique and left inferior rectus.

e. Right superior oblique and left superior rectus.

f. Right lateral rectus and left medial rectus.

A.

a. True. **b.** False. **c.** False. **d.** False. **e.** False. **f.** False.

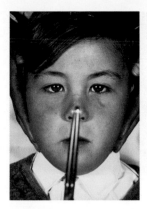

4   Q. Define the following.

a. Fusional convergence.

b. Accommodative convergence.

c. Sherrington law.

d. Hering law.

e. Horopter.

f. Panum fusional space.

A.

a. An optomotor reflex, which maintains binocular single vision, by ensuring that similar images are projected onto corresponding retinal areas or each eye. It is initiated by bitemporal retinal image disparity. **b.** It is induced by the act of accommodation as part of the synkinetic-near reflex (see above). **c.** Increased innervation to an extraocular muscle (e.g. right medial rectus) is accompanied by a reciprocal decrease in innervation to its antagonist (e.g. right lateral rectus). **d.** During any conjugate eye movement, equal and simultaneous innervation flows to the yoke muscles. **e.** An imaginary surface in space of which all points stimulate corresponding retinal elements and are therefore seen singly. **f.** A zone in front or and behind the horopter in which objects stimulate slightly non-corresponding retinal points but are perceived singly.

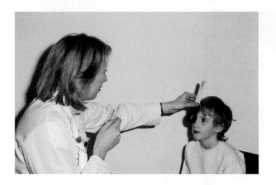

5   Q. Abnormal retinal correspondence – true or false?

a. It can be detected on the cover-uncover test (see above).

b. The fovea of one eye is paired with a non-foveal area of the deviated eye.

c. It is more frequent in small angle esotropia.

d. Objective and subjective angles are the same.

e. In harmonious abnormal retinal correspondence, the objective angle is the same as the angle of anomaly.

f. Following surgery the patient always reverts to normal retinal correspondence.

A.

a. False. **b.** True. **c.** True. **d.** False – different. **e.** True. **f.** False.

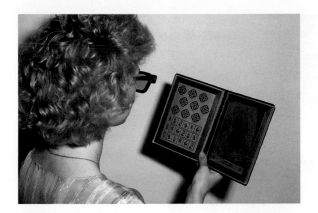

6 Q. Tests for stereopsis – answer the following.

a. What is normal stereo-acuity?

b. In the Titmus test (see above) what is the degree of disparity of the circles?

c. Of what does the TNO test consist?

d. What types of spectacles are required in the Lang test?

e. What is the degree of disparity of the Lang test?

f. Of what does the Frisby test consist?

A.

a. 60 seconds of arc. **b.** Between 800 and 40 seconds of arc. **c.** Seven plates that are viewed with red-green spectacles. **d.** Spectacles are not required. **e.** 1200 to 600 seconds of arc. **f.** Three transparent plastic plates of varying thickness each consisting of four squares of randomly distributed shapes.

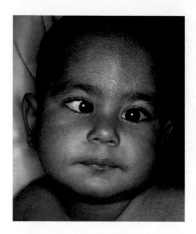

7   Q. Early-onset esotropia – true or false?

a. Presentation is within 3 months of birth.

b. Refraction is usually between +1.00 and +2.00.

c. Angle of deviation is usually small and unstable.

d. Ideally the eyes should be aligned surgically by the age of 12 months.

e. Dissociated vertical divergence is common at presentation.

f. Inferior oblique overaction may be present at presentation or may develop subsequently.

A.

a. False – within 6 months of birth. **b.** True. **c.** False – large and stable (see above). **d.** True. **e.** False – develops later. **f.** True.

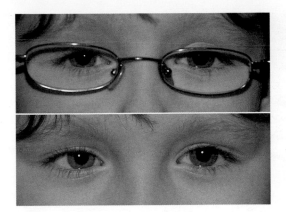

8   Q. Esotropia – true or false?

a. In refractive accommodative esotropia the AC/A ratio is high.

b. In fully accommodative refractive esotropia the deviation is eliminated with glasses.

c. In constant refractive accommodative esotropia the angle is reduced but not eliminated by full correction of hypermetropia.

d. In convergence excess non-refractive esotropia the AC/A ratio is normal and the eyes are straight for distance.

e. After the age of 8 years, refraction should be performed without cycloplegia and the maximal amount of 'plus' that can be tolerated (manifest hypermetropia) prescribed.

f. Most cases of microtropia require surgery.

A.

a. False – AC/A is normal. **b.** True (see above). **c.** True. **d.** False – AC/A is high. **e.** True. **f.** False.

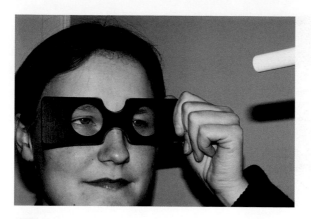

9   Q. Microtropia – true or false?

a. It may follow surgery for esotropia.

b. The deviation is 15Δ or less.

c. The deviation is worse for near than distance.

d. Anisometropia is very common.

e. Krimsky test is most useful for diagnosis.

f. Bagolini glasses (see above) show a central suppression scotoma of the deviating eye.

A.

a. True. **b.** False 8Δ or less. **c.** False. **d.** True. **e.** False. **f.** True.

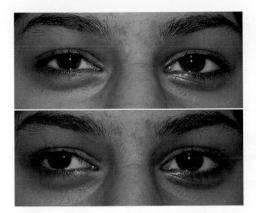

10 Q. Exotropia – true or false?

a. Constant early-onset exotropia often presents at birth.

b. Constant early-onset exotropia is usually associated with high myopia.

c. Intermittent exotropia often presents at puberty.

d. In distance intermittent exotropia the angle of deviation is greater for distance than near and increases further beyond 6 metres.

e. Secondary exotropia may follow surgery for esotropia.

f. Consecutive exotropia may develop spontaneously.

A.

a. True. **b.** False. **c.** False – at about 2 years of age. **d.** True (see above).
e. False – it occurs secondarily to a long-standing acquired lesion that impairs vision. **f.** True – if the eye is amblyopic.

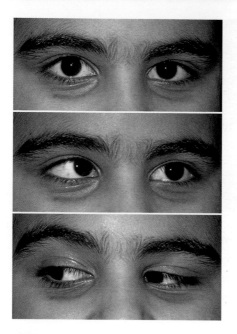

11 Q. The following occur in left Duane syndrome – true or false?

a. Restricted left abduction.

b. Normal or restricted left adduction.

c. Narrowing of the palpebral fissure on left adduction.

d. Up-shoot or down-shoot on left abduction.

e. Mild nystagmus on left abduction.

f. Deficiency of convergence of the left eye.

A. (see above)

a. True. **b.** True. **c.** True. **d.** False – adduction. **e.** False. **f.** True.

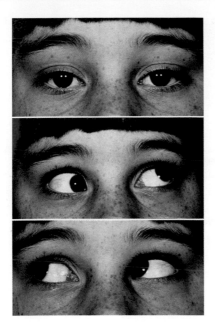

12   Q. The following occur in right Brown syndrome – true or false?

a. Binocular vision in the primary position is rare.

b. Limited right elevation on adduction.

c. Limited right elevation on abduction.

d. Left superior oblique overaction on right gaze.

e. Limitation of right adduction.

f. Positive forced duction test.

A. (see above)

a. False – it is the rule. **b.** True. **c.** False. **d.** False. **e.** False. **f.** True.

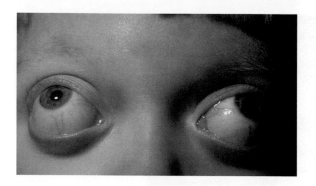

13   **Q. The following conditions may cause a 'V' pattern deviation – true or false?**

a. Fourth nerve palsy.

b. Crouzon disease.

c. Brown syndrome.

d. Duane syndrome.

e. Möbius syndrome.

f. Gradenigo syndrome.

A.

a. True. **b.** True (see above). **c.** True. **d.** False. **e.** False. **f.** False.

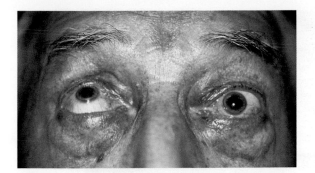

14 **Q. The following conditions are suitable for adjustable suture surgery – true or false?**

a. Old blow-out orbital floor fracture.

b. Early-onset esotropia.

c. Chronic external ophthalmoplegia.

d. Recent sixth nerve palsy.

e. Adult exotropia.

f. Thyroid myopathy.

A.

a. True. **b.** False. **c.** False. **d.** False. **e.** True. **f.** True (see above).

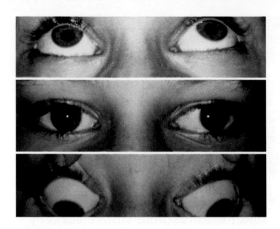

15   Q. The following may result in a chin-down position – true or false?

a. 'A' pattern exotropia.
b. 'A' pattern esotropia.
c. Myasthenia gravis.
d. Bilateral fourth nerve palsy.
e. Down-beat nystagmus.
f. Childhood hydrocephalus

A.
a. True (see above). **b.** False. **c.** False – chin-up to compensate for ptosis
d. True. **e.** True. **f.** False.

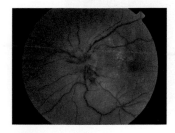

1 Q. Define the following.

a. Primary optic atrophy.

b. Secondary optic atrophy.

c. Optic neuritis.

d. Retrobulbar neuritis.

e. Papillitis.

f. Neuroretinitis.

A.

a. This occurs without antecedent swelling of the optic nerve head and may be caused by lesions affecting the visual pathways from the retrolaminar portion of the optic nerve to the lateral geniculate body. **b.** This is preceded by swelling of the optic nerve head. **c.** This is an Inflammatory, infective or demyelinating process affecting the optic nerve. **d.** This involves the retrolaminar part of the optic nerve and is characterized by a normal appearing optic disc. **e.** This is characterized by variable hyperaemia and oedema of the optic disc which may be associated with peripapillary flame-shaped haemorrhages. **f.** This is characterized by papillitis in association with inflammation of the retinal nerve fibre layer and a macular star figure (see above).

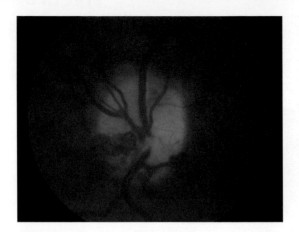

2 **Q. Match the optic neuropathy (a–f) with the appropriate underlying cause (i–vi).**

a. Primary optic atrophy.

b. Secondary optic atrophy.

c. Retrobulbar neuritis.

d. Papillitis.

e. Neuroretinitis.

f. Opticociliary shunts (see above).

i. Multiple sclerosis (MS).

ii. Pituitary adenoma.

iii. Cat scratch disease.

iv. Optic nerve sheath meningioma.

v. Papilloedema.

vi. Bilateral visual loss in children.

A.

a. & **ii**; b. & **v**; c. & **i**; d. & **vi**; e. & **iii**; f. & **iv**.

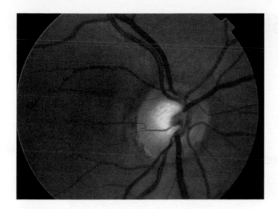

3   Q. Optic neuritis in MS – true or false?

a. 15–20% of MS patients present with retrobulbar neuritis and a normal fundus (see above).

b. The overall 10-year risk of developing MS following an acute episode of optic neuritis is 50%.

c. Approximately 75% of patients recover visual acuity to 6/9 or better.

d. Vision does not usually improve if visual acuity is reduced to 'light perception' during an attack of optic neuritis.

e. Treatment speeds up recovery but does not influence the eventual visual outcome.

f. Treatment with intravenous interferon beta-1a at the first episode of optic neuritis may be beneficial in reducing the subsequent development of MS.

A.

a. True. **b.** False – risk is 38%. **c.** True. **d.** False. **e.** True.
f. False – intramuscular.

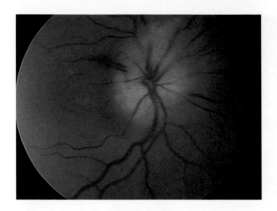

4   Q. Non-arteritic anterior ischaemic optic neuropathy – true or false?

a. It typically affects patients over the age of 70 years.

b. Hypertension is a common association.

c. The disc is pale and swollen and often shows a few splinter-shaped haemorrhages.

d. Involvement of the fellow eye is 15% after 5 years.

e. Aspirin usually prevents involvement of the fellow eye.

f. Recurrence in the same eye is uncommon.

A.

a. False – between the age of 55 and 70 years. **b.** True. **c.** True (see above). **d.** True. **e.** False. **f.** True.

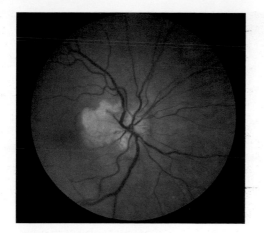

5   **Q. Arteritic anterior ischaemic optic neuropathy – true or false?**

a. At presentation the majority of patients do not have systemic symptoms of giant-cell arteritis.

b. Transient visual obscurations may precede visual loss.

c. It may be associated with simultaneous occlusion of a cilioretinal artery.

d. Bilateral simultaneous involvement is common.

e. With early treatment vision recovers in 25% of cases.

f. Steroid therapy should not be started prior to temporal artery biopsy.

A.

a. False – 20%. **b.** True. **c.** True (see above). **d.** False. **e.** False – recovery is rare. **f.** False.

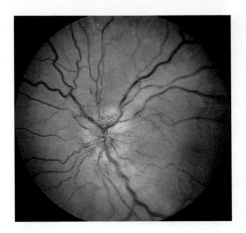

6   Q. Leber hereditary optic neuropathy – true or false?

a. It typically affects young males.

b. Presentation is with bilateral simultaneous visual loss.

c. Dilated capillaries on the disc surface are characteristic.

d. Pupillary responses to light may be brisk despite severe involvement.

e. Systemic steroids are effective in 50% of cases if instituted during the first week.

f. Prognosis is more favourable in patients with DNA mutation 11778.

A.

a. True. **b.** False. **c.** True (see above). **d.** True. **e.** False. **f.** False – it is less favourable.

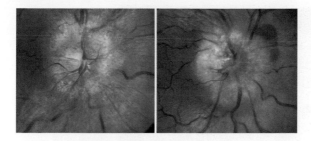

7   Q. Papilloedema – answer the following.

a. What is papilloedema?

b. What is the opening CSF pressure on lumbar puncture in adults?

c. What is the cause of horizontal diplopia in patients with raised intracranial pressure?

d. What is the mechanism of non-communicating hydrocephalus?

e. Is papilloedema present in all patients with raised intracranial pressure?

f. What is the eventual consequence of unrelieved papilloedema?

A.

a. Bilateral swelling of the optic nerve head secondary to raised intracranial pressure (see above). **b.** <210 mm of water. **c.** Sixth nerve palsy caused by stretching of one or both sixth nerves over the petrous tip as a result of downward displacement of the brain stem. **d.** Obstruction to CSF flow in the ventricular system or at the exit foramina of the fourth ventricle. **e.** No. **f.** Secondary optic atrophy

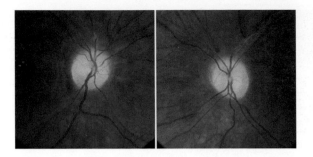

8   Q. Idiopathic intracranial hypertension – true or false?

a. It typically affects young overweight women.

b. The mortality rate is 25%.

c. Transient visual 'blackouts' are characteristic.

d. Optic-nerve fenestration does not prevent visual loss from bilateral secondary optic atrophy (see above).

e. Neuroimaging shows dilated ventricles.

f. Diuretics may relieve headache.

A.

a. True. **b.** False. **c.** True. **d.** False. **e.** False. **f.** True.

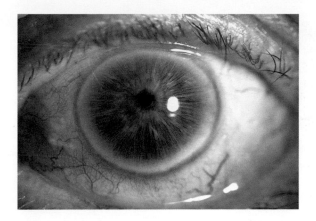

9

Q. Match the pupil (a–f) with the appropriate association (i–vi).

a. Amaurotic pupil.

b. Marcus Gunn pupil.

c. Argyll Robertson pupil (see above).

d. Adie pupil.

e. Horner syndrome.

f. Wernicke hemianopic pupil.

i. Positive swinging flashlight test.

ii. Optic tract lesion.

iii. No light perception.

iv. Ptosis and miosis.

v. Tonic accommodation.

vi. Bilateral light-near dissociation.

A.

a. & **iii**; b. & **i**; c. & **vi**; d. & **v**; e. & **iv**; f. & **ii**.

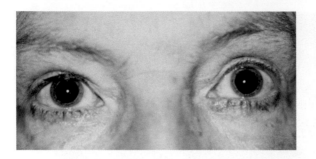

10 Q. Horner syndrome – true or false?

a. Reduced ipsilateral sweating may occur but only if the lesion is above the superior cervical ganglion.

b. Pancoast tumour may damage the second pre-ganglionic neuron.

c. The ciliospinal centre of Budge is between C8 and T2.

d. Cocaine 4% dilates a Horner pupil but not a normal pupil.

e. Hydroxyamfetamine 1% dilates a normal pupil and a preganglionic Horner pupil.

f. Adrenaline 1:1000 will dilate neither a normal pupil nor a preganglionic Horner pupil.

A.

a. False – below. **b.** True. **c.** True. **d.** False – reverse applies. **e.** True (see above). **f.** True.

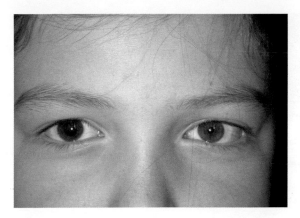

11 Q. Pupillary abnormalities – true or false?

a. An afferent conduction defect can only be caused by a lesion of the optic nerve.

b. A long-standing Adie pupil may become small.

c. Adie pupil will constrict to 0.125% pilocarpine but the normal pupil will not.

d. An amaurotic pupil is slightly smaller than the normal pupil.

e. In motor involvement the affected pupil may be larger than the normal pupil.

f. Cluster headaches may cause a central (first order neuron) Horner.

A.

a. False. **b.** True – 'little old Adie'. **c.** True (see above). **d.** False.

e. True. **f.** False – post-ganglionic (third order neuron) Horner.

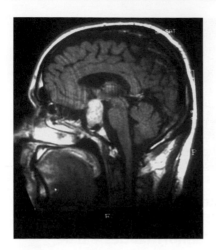

12   Q. Chiasmal disorders – true or false?

a. Absence of a visual field defect does not exclude a pituitary tumour.

b. Optic atrophy is present in the majority of patients with field defects caused by pituitary tumours.

c. Craniopharyngiomas tend to cause bilateral inferior temporal visual field defects.

d. MR in the axial plane is optimal for demonstrating sellar contents.

e. Solid craniopharyngiomas are hyperintense on T1-weighted images on MR.

f. Pituitary adenomas enhance strongly with gadolinium on MR.

A.

a. True. **b.** False – 50%. **c.** True. **d.** False – coronal. **e.** False – isointense.
f. True (see above).

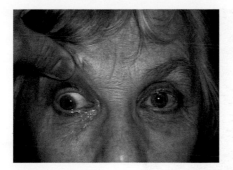

13 Q. Third cranial nerve – answer the following.

a. What are the features of Weber syndrome?

b. Which muscles are innervated by the inferior division?

c. What is the location of the pupillomotor fibres?

d. What is the most common cause of sudden painful third nerve palsy with pupil involvement?

e. What are the most common causes of pupil-sparing third nerve palsy?

f. When should surgery be considered in a third nerve palsy?

A.

a. Third nerve palsy (see above) and a contralateral hemiparesis. **b.** Medial rectus, the inferior rectus and the inferior oblique muscles. **c.** Superficial superomedial part of the nerve. **d.** Aneurysm at the junction of the posterior communicating artery, at its junction with the internal carotid artery. **e.** Hypertension and diabetes. **f.** Only after all spontaneous improvement has ceased.

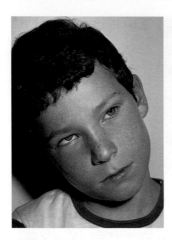

14   Q. Fourth cranial nerve – true or false?

a. It is the only cranial nerve to emerge from the dorsal aspect of the brain.

b. The fourth nerve nucleus innervates the ipsilateral superior oblique muscle.

c. Congenital lesions may not become apparent until adult life.

d. Traumatic lesions are frequently bilateral.

e. The compensatory head posture involves contralateral head tilt, contralateral face turn and chin down.

f. Bielschowsky test shows increase of hypertropia on contralateral head tilt.

A.

a. True. **b.** False – contralateral superior oblique muscle. **c.** True. **d.** True.
e. True. **f.** False – ipsilateral head tilt (see above).

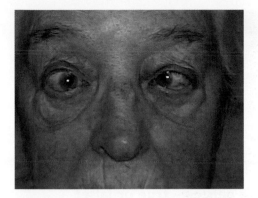

15   Q. Sixth cranial nerve – true or false?

a. Isolated sixth nerve palsy is never nuclear in origin.

b. Millard–Gubler syndrome involves the fasciculus of the sixth nerve as it passes through the pyramidal tract.

c. Foville syndrome may be associated with Horner syndrome.

d. Sixth nerve palsy (see above) may occur in migrainous neuralgia.

e. Horizontal diplopia due to sixth nerve palsy is the first sign of acoustic neuroma.

f. Aneurysms seldom affect the sixth nerve.

A.

a. True. **b.** True. **c.** True. **d.** False. **e.** False – it is diminished corneal sensation. **f.** True.

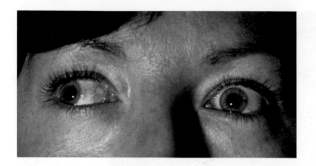

16   Q. Gaze palsies – true or false?

a. Are characterized by absence of diplopia and normal vestibulo-ocular reflexes.

b. A lesion involving the pontine paramedian reticular formation (PPRF) gives rise to ipsilateral horizontal gaze palsy with inability to look in the direction of the lesion.

c. A lesion of the medial longitudinal fasciculus (MLF) is characterized by defective ipsilateral adduction and ataxic nystagmus of the contralateral eye.

d. In combined lesions involving the PPRF and MLF on the same side, the only residual movement is adduction of the contralateral eye, which also exhibits ataxic nystagmus.

e. In a lesion of the MLF, convergence is usually intact if the lesion is discrete.

f. MS is an important cause of Parinaud syndrome in children.

A.

a. True. **b.** True. **c.** True (see above). **d.** False – abduction. **e.** True.
f. False.

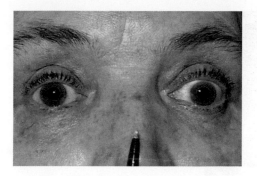

17 Q. Parinaud dorsal midbrain syndrome is characterized by – true or false?

a. Large pupils.

b. Light-near dissociation.

c. Mild bilateral ptosis.

d. Supranuclear downgaze palsy.

e. Paralysis of convergence.

f. Convergence-retraction nystagmus with vertical saccades.

A.

a. True. **b.** True. **c.** False – lid retraction. **d.** False – upgaze palsy. **e.** True (see above). **f.** True.

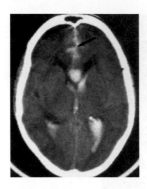

18 **Q. Intracranial aneurysms – answer the following.**

a. Describe the circle of Willis.

b. What is the most common complication?

c. What is Terson syndrome?

d. How may an aneurysm mimic a pituitary tumour?

e. What is the 'gold standard' investigation of a small aneurysm prior to surgery?

f. How are aneurysms treated?

A.

a. The anterior cerebral arteries are connected by the anterior communicating artery. The middle and posterior cerebral arteries are connected by the posterior communicating artery. This anastomosis forms the circle of Willis, which lies in the subarachnoid space on the ventral surface of the brain. **b.** Rupture giving rise to subarachnoid haemorrhage (see above).
c. A combination of intraocular haemorrhage and subarachnoid haemorrhage secondary to aneurysmal rupture. **d.** An aneurysm arising from the intracavernous part of the internal carotid artery may erode into the sella and mimic a pituitary tumour. **e.** Conventional intra-arterial angiography. **f.** By placing a clip around the neck of the aneurysm or, less frequently, the insertion of soft metallic coils within the lumen.

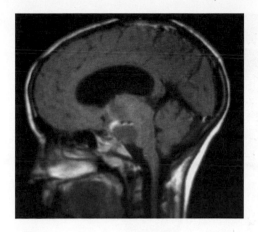

19 **Q. Match the nystagmus (a–f) with the appropriate association (i–vi).**

a. Sensory deprivation nystagmus.

b. Downbeat nystagmus.

c. Convergence-retraction nystagmus.

d. See-saw nystagmus of Maddox.

e. Ataxic nystagmus.

f. Latent nystagmus.

i. Pinealoma.

ii. MS.

iii. Pituitary adenoma.

iv. Early-onset esotropia.

v. Leber amaurosis.

vi. Arnold–Chiari malformation (see above).

A.

a. & **v**; **b.** & **vi**; **c.** & **i**; **d.** & **iii**; **e.** & **ii**; **f.** & **iv**.

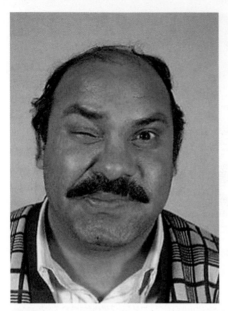

20 **Q. Match the eponymous condition (a–f) with the appropriate association (i–vi).**

a. Charles Bonnet syndrome.

b. L' Hermitte sign.

c. Anton syndrome.

d. Uhthoff phenomenon.

e. Miller–Fisher syndrome.

f. Meige syndrome.

i. Electric shock sensation on neck flexion.

ii. Blepharospasm (see above).

iii. Visual hallucinations.

iv. Bilateral ophthalmoplegia and facial palsy.

v. Visual deterioration on exposure to heat.

vi. Denial of blindness.

A.

a. & iii; b. & i; c. & vi; d. & v; e. & iv; f. & ii.

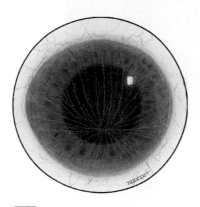

1 Q. Vortex keratopathy – true or false?

a. Severity of involvement is usually asymmetrical.

b. It may cause moderate impairment of vision.

c. Its appearance is related to the dose and duration of chloroquine therapy.

d. It occasionally develops for no apparent reason.

e. It is rare in patients on amiodarone.

f. It may occur in patients on long-term chlorpromazine therapy.

A.

a. False. **b.** False. **c.** False. **d.** False. **e.** False. **f.** False.

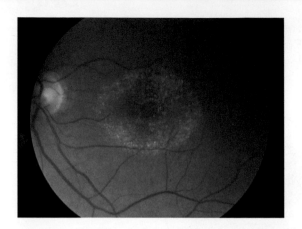

2 **Q. Match the drug (a–f) with the appropriate association (i–vi).**

a. Gentamicin.

b. Rifabutin.

c. Chloroquine.

d. Systemic steroids.

e. Tamoxifen.

f. Interferon alpha.

i. Bull's eye maculopathy.

ii. Macular infarction.

iii. Acute anterior uveitis.

iv. Fine, superficial, yellow, crystalline retinal deposits at the posterior pole.

v. Posterior subcapsular lens opacities.

vi. Cotton-wool spots and intraretinal haemorrhages.

A.

a. & **ii**; **b.** & **iii**; **c.** & **i**; **d.** & **v**; **e.** & **iv** (see above); **f.** & **vi**.

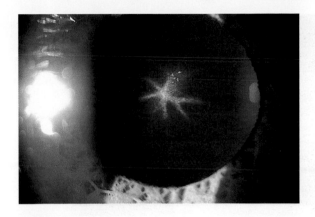

3 Q. Drugs that may cause lens opacities or deposits – true or false?

a. Busulfan.

b. Tamoxifen.

c. Ciclosporin.

d. Thioridazine.

e. Chlorpromazine.

f. Allopurinol.

A.

a. True. **b.** False. **c.** False. **d.** False. **e.** True (see above). **f.** True.

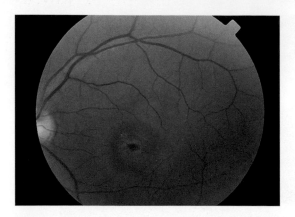

4   **Q. Ocular drug toxicity – true or false?**

a. Hydroxychloroquine maculopathy (see above) is rare.

b. Amiodarone optic neuropathy is dose-related.

c. Chlorpromazine may cause subtle corneal deposits.

d. Visual field defects caused by vigabatrin are reversible on cessation of treatment.

e. Gold may cause band keratopathy.

f. Ethambutol may cause optic neuropathy.

A.

a. True. **b.** False. **c.** True. **d.** False. **e.** False. **f.** True.

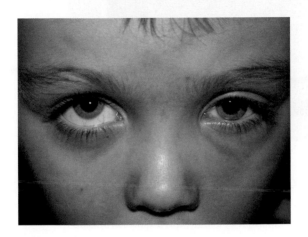

1   Q. Orbital fractures – true or false?

a. Pure blow-out fracture does not involve the orbital rim.

b. Ocular damage is uncommon in floor blow-out fractures.

c. Enophthalmos is an indication for urgent repair of a floor blow-out fracture.

d. Diplopia may be caused by entrapment of the inferior rectus muscle.

e. Medial blow-out fracture often causes 'panda eyes'.

f. Large roof fractures manifest pulsation of the globe associated with a bruit due to transmission of CSF pulsation.

A.

a. True. **b.** True. **c.** False. **d.** True (see above). **e.** False – refers to roof fracture. **f.** False – bruit is absent.

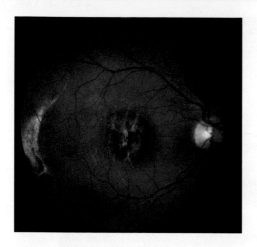

2   Q. Blunt trauma – true or false?

a. Tears in Descemet membrane are usually horizontal.

b. Corneal abrasions heal more quickly when the eye is patched.

c. Most hyphaemas are innocuous and transient.

d. Vossius ring is a subcapsular lens opacity.

e. Commotio retinae rarely gives rise to macular hole formation.

f. Choroidal ruptures are solitary.

A.

a. False – vertical. **b.** False. **c.** True. **d.** False – consists of iris pigment.
e. True. **f.** False (see above).

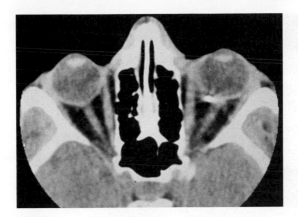

3   Q. Penetrating trauma – true or false?

a. Intraocular fragment of shrapnel will cause more damage than an air gun pellet.

b. CT with axial and coronal cuts is used to detect and localize metallic intraocular foreign bodies.

c. Siderosis may give rise to heterochromia iridis.

d. Electroretinography in siderosis manifests progressive attenuation of the a-wave over time.

e. Chalcosis may cause an endophthalmitis-like reaction.

f. The vast majority of cases of sympathetic ophthalmitis present within 3 months of injury.

A.

a. False – reverse applies. **b.** True (see above). **c.** True. **d.** False – b-wave. **e.** True. **f.** False – within the first year.

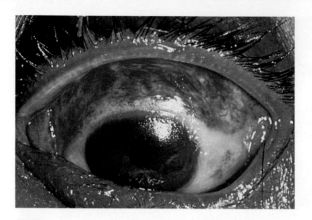

4   Q. Chemical injuries – true or false?

a. Acids tend to penetrate deeper than alkalis.

b. Severity of limbal ischaemia (see above) is an important prognostic factor.

c. Ascorbic acid is used topically and systemically.

d. Citric acid reduces the intensity of the inflammatory response.

e. Topical steroids may be used initially but must be tailed off after 14 days.

f. Keratoplasty should be delayed for at least 6 months and preferably longer to allow maximal resolution of inflammation.

A.

a. False – reverse applies. **b.** True. **c.** True. **d.** True. **e.** False – must be tailed off after 7–10 days. **f.** True.

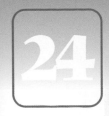
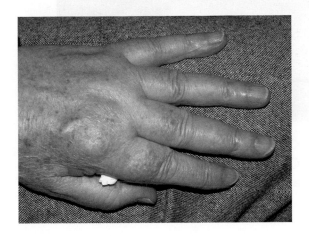

1 Q. Rheumatoid arthritis – answer the following.

a. Which are the most commonly involved joints?
b. What is the incidence of uveitis?
c. What is the most common ocular manifestation?
d. What is the most serious ocular manifestation?
e. What is the least common ocular manifestation?
f. What is the most serious systemic complication?

A.

a. Small joints of the hands (see above). **b.** Nil. **c.** Keratoconjunctivitis sicca. **d.** Posterior scleritis. **e.** Acquired superior oblique tendon sheath syndrome. **f.** Secondary amyloidosis.

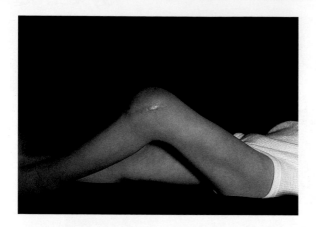

2   **Q. Juvenile idiopathic arthritis (JIA) – answer the following.**

a. What is JIA?

b. What are the most commonly involved joints?

c. What is the female to male ratio?

d. What is polyarticular JIA?

e. What percentage of patients present with paulyarticular JIA?

f. What is the main ocular manisfestation?

A.

a. Sero-negative arthritis of unknown aetiology developing prior to the age of 16 years. **b.** Knees (see above). **c.** 3:2. **d.** Involvement of five or more joints. **e.** 60%. **f.** Chronic anterior uveitis.

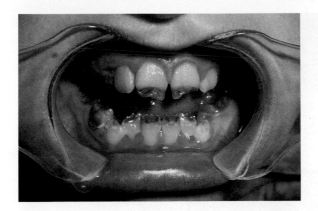

3   Q. Sjögren syndrome – true or false?

a. It is an autoimmune disease characterized by polymorphonuclear infiltration of lacrimal and salivary glands.

b. Severe xerostomia may cause dental caries.

c. Primary Sjögren syndrome typically affects elderly men.

d. Most patients with primary Sjögren syndrome carry antinuclear antibodies.

e. Systemic lupus erythematosus is the most common cause of secondary Sjögren syndrome.

f. Secondary Sjögren syndrome occasionally may be associated with liver disease.

A.

a. False – lymphocytic infiltration. **b.** True (see above). **c.** False – women.
d. True. **e.** False – rheumatoid arthritis. **f.** True – biliary cirrhosis.

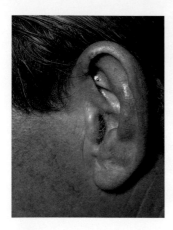

4   **Q. True or false?**

a. In Reiter syndrome uveitis is more common than conjunctivitis.
b. MS is associated with chronic anterior uveitis.
c. Wegener granulomatosis may cause nasolacrimal duct obstruction.
d. Polyarteritis nodosa may be associated with Cogan syndrome.
e. Keratoconjunctivitis sicca is rare in psoriatic arthritis.
f. Relapsing polychondritis (see above) is an important cause of intractable scleritis.

A.

a. False – reverse applies. **b.** False – intermediate uveitis. **c.** True. **d.** True.
e. True. **f.** True.

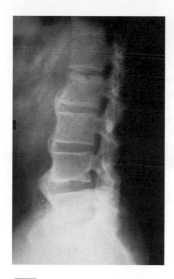

5   Q. Ankylosing spondylitis – true or false?

a. In children it may present with lower limb arthritis.

b. The majority of patients are positive for HLA-B27.

c. Acute anterior uveitis occurs in 45% of cases.

d. Non-necrotizing scleritis occurs in about 10% of cases.

e. Radiological changes (see above) often antedate clinical symptoms.

f. Treatment involves systemic steroids.

A.

a. True. **b.** True. **c.** False – 25%. **d.** False – it is very rare. **e.** True.
f. False.

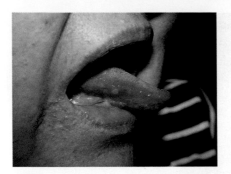

6   **Q. The following occur in Reiter syndrome – true or false?**

a. Painful aphthous stomatitis (see above).

b. Dysentery.

c. Nail dystrophy.

d. Sero-positive arthropathy.

e. Calcaneal spur.

f. Aortic stenosis.

A.

a. False – painless. **b.** True. **c.** True. **d.** False – sero-negative. **e.** True.

f. False – incompetence.

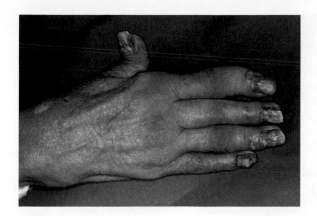

7 Q. Psoriatic arthritis – true or false?

a. About 15% of patients with psoriasis develop arthritis
(see above).

b. It typically affects young men.

c. It may affect children.

d. A small minority of patients develop Crohn disease.

e. Uveitis is less common than in Reiter syndrome.

f. Sacroiliitis does not occur.

A.

a. False – 7%. **b.** False – affects both sexes equally. **c.** True. **d.** False.
e. True. **f.** False.

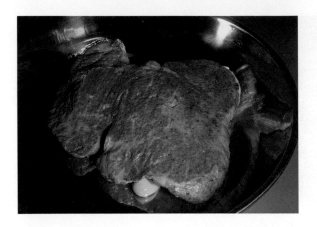

8   Q. Inflammatory bowel disease – true or false?

a. Ulcerative colitis may be associated with liver disease
(see above).

b. Some patients with Reiter syndrome develop ulcerative colitis.

c. Anterior uveitis is uncommon in ulcerative colitis unless it is
associated with sacroiliitis.

d. Most patients with Crohn disease do not have ocular
manifestations.

e. Patients with longstanding Crohn disease carry an increased
risk of carcinoma of the caecum.

f. Whipple disease is caused by infection.

A.

a. True.   **b.** False.   **c.** True.   **d.** True.   **e.** False – ulcerative colitis.   **f.** True.

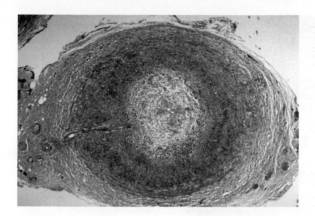

9   Q. Giant cell arteritis – answer the following.

a. What percentage of patients has a normal ESR?

b. Why are intracranial arteries spared?

c. What are the features of polymyalgia rheumatica?

d. Which symptom is virtually pathognomonic?

e. What length of temporal artery is required for adequate biopsy (see above)?

f. What determines the duration of steroid therapy?

A.

a. 20%. **b.** Because they contain little elastic tissue. **c.** Pain and stiffness in proximal muscle groups (typically the shoulders), which are characteristically worse in the morning and after exertion. **d.** Jaw claudication. **e.** 2.5 cm. **f.** Symptoms and the level of the ESR or C-reactive protein.

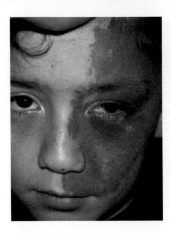

10   **Q. Match the syndrome (a–f) with the most appropriate ophthalmic manifestation (i–vi).**

a. Sturge–Weber syndrome (see above).

b. Marfan syndrome.

c. Stickler syndrome.

d. Grönblad–Strandberg syndrome.

e. Hermansky–Pudlak syndrome.

f. Kearns–Sayre syndrome.

i. Angioid streaks.

ii. Diffuse choroidal haemangioma.

iii. Ocular albinism.

iv. Pigmentary retinopathy.

v. Radial lattice degeneration.

vi. Ectopia lentis.

A.

a. & **ii**; **b.** & **vi**; **c.** & **v**; **d.** & **i**; **e.** & **iii**; **f.** & **iv**.

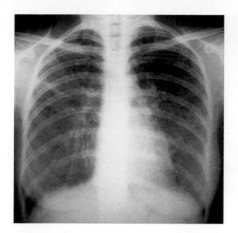

11 Q. Sarcoidosis – answer the following.

a. What is Löfgren syndrome?

b. What is Heerfordt syndrome (uveoparotid fever)?

c. What are the radiological features of stage 3 pulmonary involvement?

d. What is erythema nodosum?

e. What is lupus pernio?

f. What is the normal serum ACE level in healthy adults?

A.

a. Combination of erythema nodosum and bilateral hilar lymphadenopathy, often accompanied by fever and/or arthritis. **b.** Combination of uveitis, parotid gland enlargement, fever and often facial nerve palsy. **c.** Diffuse parenchymal reticulonodular infiltration without hilar adenopathy (see above). **d.** Tender erythematous plaques typically involving the knees and shins and occasionally the thighs and forearms. **e.** Indurated, violaceous lesions involving exposed parts of the body such as the nose, cheeks, fingers or ears. **f.** 32.1 +/- 8.5 IU.

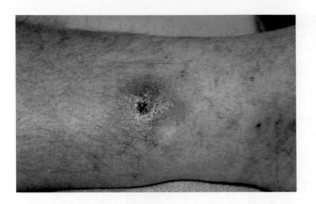

12 **Q. Behçet syndrome – answer the following.**

a. What is the HLA association?

b. Are ocular complications more common in males or females?

c. What is the usual interval between aphthous stomatitis and the onset of eye disease?

d. What is a positive pathergy test?

e. What are the characteristics of arthritis?

f. What is the most common neurological manifestation?

A.

a. HLA-B51. **b.** Males. **c.** 2 years. **d.** Formation of a pustule 24–48 hours after a prick with a sterile needle (see above). **e.** It is mild and involves a few large joints, particularly the knees. **f.** Brain stem involvement.

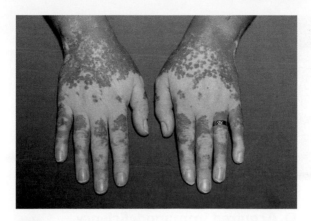

13 Q. Vogt–Koyanagi–Harada syndrome – true or false?

a. It is associated with HLA-DR1 and HLA-DR3.

b. Possible trigger factors include cutaneous injury or a viral infection which may lead to sensitization of melanosomes.

c. It is common in dark-skinned individuals.

d. Vogt–Koyanagi syndrome is characterized mainly by vitiligo and anterior uveitis.

e. Harada disease in characterized by which neurological features and bilateral tractional retinal detachments.

f. Mortality is high if treatment is delayed.

A.

a. False – HLA-DR1 and HLA-DR4. **b.** True – sensitization to melanocytes. **c.** True. **d.** True (see above). **e.** False – exudative retinal detachments. **f.** False.

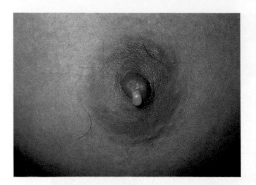

14   Q. Acquired immunodeficiency syndrome – true or false?

a. The virus can be transmitted via breast milk (see above).

b. Indications for commencement of anti-HIV therapy include CD4+T-lymphocyte count <500/mm^3.

c. 'Seroconversion' may take 3 months or longer to occur following exposure to the virus.

d. Drug treatment is with 'highly active antiretroviral therapy' (HAART), which involves 2 nucleoside reverse transcriptase inhibitors with either a non-nucleoside reverse transcriptase inhibitor or 1 or 2 protease inhibitors.

e. Zidovudine is a protease inhibitor.

f. Nevirapine is a non-nucleoside reverse transcriptase inhibitor.

A.

a. True. **b.** False – <300/mm^3. **c.** True. **d.** True. **e.** False – it is a nucleoside reverse transcriptase inhibitor. **f.** True.

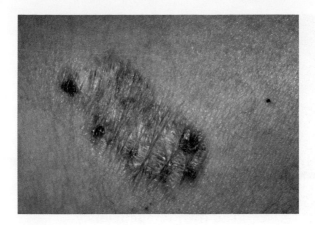

15 Q. Tuberculosis (TB) – true or false?

a. The tubercle bacillus is a motile, non-sporing, anaerobic rod.

b. Human immunodeficiency virus increases the risk of developing TB.

c. In latent TB the Mantoux test is negative.

d. A negative Mantoux test may occur in patients with miliary TB.

e. Most patients with ocular involvement have miliary disease.

f. It may cause Parinaud oculoglandular syndrome.

A.

a. False – it is non-motile and aerobic. **b.** True. **c.** False – positive (see above). **d.** True. **e.** False. **f.** True.

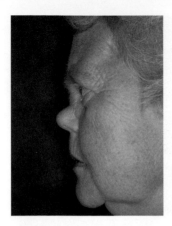

16 Q. Syphilis – true or false?

a. The spirochaete does not live in culture.

b. Without treatment the primary chancre may persist for 2 to 6 months.

c. Anterior uveitis usually occurs during the primary stage.

d. Condylomata lata occur in the tertiary stage.

e. The latent stage lasts a few months.

f. A saddle-shaped nose (see above) is typical of gummatous involvement.

A.

a. True. **b.** False – 2–6 weeks. **c.** False – secondary and tertiary stages.
d. False – secondary stage. **e.** False – may last several years. **f.** False – occurs in congenital disease.

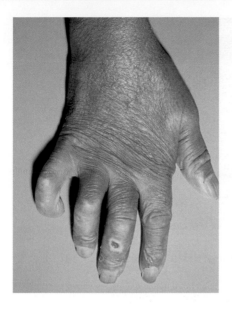

17 Q. Leprosy – true or false?

a. It is a chronic vasculitis caused by an intracellular acid-fast bacillus *Mycobacterium leprae*.

b. The skin appears to be the most likely portal of entry.

c. Leonine facies occurs in lepromatous leprosy.

d. Tuberculoid leprosy is confined to the skin and peripheral nerve.

e. 'Claw hand' (see above) occurs in tuberculoid leprosy.

f. The leprin test is negative in lepromatous leprosy.

A.

a. False – a chronic granulomatous disease. **b.** False – upper respiratory tract. **c.** True. **d.** True. **e.** False – lepromatous leprosy. **f.** True.

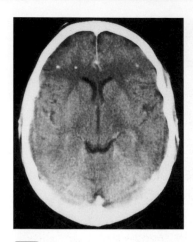

18 Q. Toxoplasmosis – true or false?

a. The cat is intermediate host.

b. Sporozoites are inactive and are contained within tissue cysts.

c. Tachyzoites cause tissue destruction and inflammation.

d. MR in congenital toxoplasmosis may show cerebral calcification.

e. Most cases of acquired toxoplasmosis are characterized by a transient fever and lymphadenopathy.

f. In AIDS the most common manifestation of acquired toxoplasmosis is an intracerebral space occupying lesion which resembles a cerebral abscess on MR.

A.

a. False – definitive host. **b.** False – refers to bradyzoites. **c.** True.
d. False – CT may show calcification (see above). **e.** False – most are
subclinical. **f.** True.

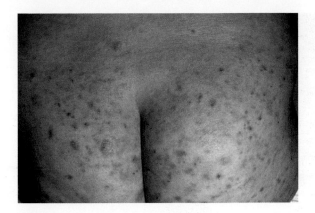

19 Q. Systemic infections – true or false?

a. About 80% of puppies between the ages of 2 and 6 months are infested with *Toxocara canis*.

b. Ocular toxocariasis is not associated with systemic involvement.

c. The most common early manifestation of onchocerciasis are subcutaneous nodules (onchocercomas).

d. Cryptococcosis primarily involves the central nervous system.

e. Cysticercosis often involves the liver and spleen.

f. Nocardia typically causes non-caseating granulomatous inflammation.

A.

a. True. **b.** True. **c.** False – pruritic papules (see above). **d.** True. **e.** False – lungs, muscles and brain. **f.** False – it causes suppurative necrosis and abscess formation.

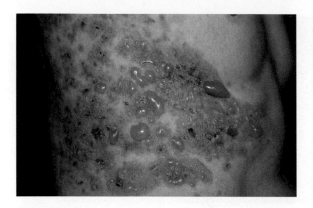

20 Q. Mucous membrane pemphigoid – true or false?

a. Men are affected more commonly than women.

b. The genitalia may be occasionally affected.

c. Patients who present before the age of 60 years tend to have more severe ocular and systemic involvement.

d. Conjunctival disease is more common in patients with skin lesions (see above) than with oral involvement.

e. Conjunctival disease never occurs in isolation.

f. Generalized skin involvement is uncommon.

A.

a. False – reverse applies. **b.** True. **c.** True. **d.** False – the reverse applies.
e. False. **f.** True.

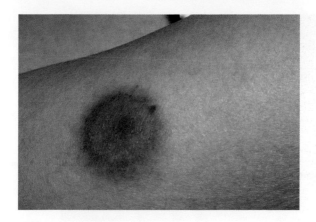

21 Q. Stevens–Johnson syndrome – true or false?

a. Males are affected more often than females.

b. Mean age at onset is 45 years.

c. The precipitating factor is usually apparent.

d. Presentation is with fever, malaise, sore throat, and possibly cough and arthralgia which may last up to 14 days before the appearance of mucocutaneous lesions.

e. Blisters are usually transient but may be widespread and associated with haemorrhage and necrosis.

f. 'Target' lesions (see above) usually evolve into a generalized erythematous rash.

A.

a. True. **b.** False – 25 years. **c.** False – only in 50%. **d.** True. **e.** True.
f. False – reverse applies.

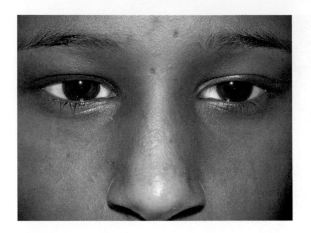

22   Q. Ocular associations of atopic eczema – true or false?

a. Madarosis.

b. Seborrhoeic blepharitis.

c. Chronic keratoconjunctivitis.

d. Keratoglobus.

e. Cataract.

f. Retinal detachment.

A.

a. True (see above). **b.** False – staphylococcal. **c.** True. **d.** False – keratoconus. **e.** True. **f.** True.

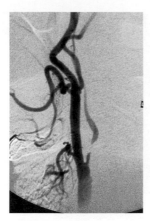

23 Q. Carotid stenosis – answer the following.

a. What is carotid stenosis?

b. What is the most common presenting symptom?

c. What is the composition of emboli arising from carotid stenosis?

d. What is the most serious complication?

e. Which antiplatelet drugs may be used?

f. What are the indications for carotid endarterectomy?

A.

a. Atheromatous narrowing and often ulceration, at the bifurcation of the common carotid artery. **b.** Transient ischaemic attacks. **c.** Fibrin-platelet (white emboli) and cholesterol (Hollenhorst) plaques. **d.** Stroke. **e.** Antiplatelet drugs are aspirin, dipyridamole (Persantin) and clopidogrel (Plavix). **f.** Carotid endarterectomy is indicated in patients with symptomatic stenosis greater than 70% (see above).

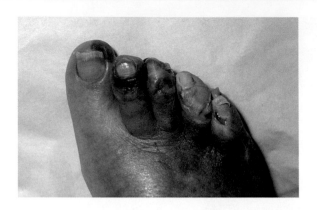

24   Q. Diabetes mellitus – answer the following.

a. What is the postulated pathogenesis of type 1 diabetes?

b. What is the upper limit of random blood glucose?

c. What is the normal range of glycosylated haemoglobin?

d. What is the characteristic distribution of sensory neuropathy?

e. What is necrobiosis lipoidica?

f. What is the pathogenesis of 'diabetic foot' (see above)?

A.

a. Autoimmune destruction of pancreatic islet cells. **b.** 10.00 mmol/ml.
c. 4–8%. **d.** 'Glove and stocking' distribution. **e.** Waxy plaques with
irregular margins and shiny centres involving the shins. **f.** Combination
of sensory neuropathy and vascular insufficiency often associated with
infection.

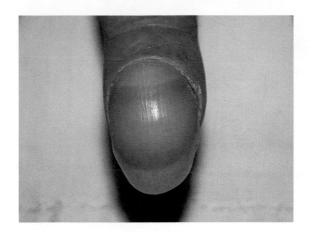

25 Q. Thyrotoxicosis – answer the following.

a. What is Graves disease?

b. What are thyroid acropachy?

c. What is pretibial myxoedema?

d. What thyroid function tests may be performed?

e. What cardiac arrhythmias may be present?

f. What are the medical treatment options?

A.

a. Most common subtype of hyperthyroidism in which IgG antibodies bind to thyroid-stimulating hormone (TSH) receptors in the thyroid gland and stimulate secretion of thyroid hormones. b. Finger clubbing (see above). c. Infiltrative dermopathy characterized by raised plaques on the anterior aspect of the legs, extending on to the dorsum of the foot. d. Serum T3, T4, TSH, thyroxine-binding globulin (TBG) and thyroid-stimulating immunoglobulin (TSI). e. Sinus tachycardia, atrial fibrillation and premature ventricular beats. f. Carbimazole, propylthiouracil, propranolol and radioactive iodine.

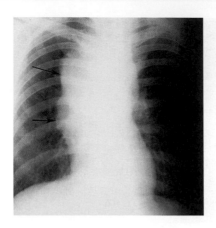

26 Q. Myasthenia gravis – answer the following.

a. What is the pathogenesis?

b. What are the main types?

c. What are the most common presenting features?

d. What percentage of patients has thymoma (see above)?

e. When performing the edrophonium test what is the test dose and the remaining dose, provided there is no hypersensitivity?

f. What drugs can be used to treat myasthenia?

A.

a. An autoimmune disease in which antibodies mediate damage and destruction of acetylcholine receptors in striated muscle. **b.** Ocular, bulbar and generalized. **c.** Ptosis and diplopia. **d.** 10%. **e.** The test dose is 0.2 ml (2 mg) and the remaining dose is 0.8 ml (8 mg). **f.** Anticholinesterase drugs (pyridostigmine, neostigmine), steroids and immunosuppressive agents (azathioprine, ciclosporin).

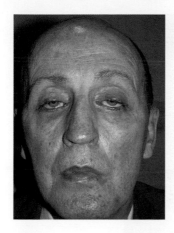

27 Q. The following may occur in myotonic dystrophy – true or false?

a. Iris heterochromia.

b. Ptosis.

c. Light-near dissociation.

d. Pigmentary glaucoma.

e. Pattern macular dystrophy.

f. Ophthalmoplegia.

A.

a. False. **b.** True (see above). **c.** True. **d.** False. **e.** True. **f.** True.

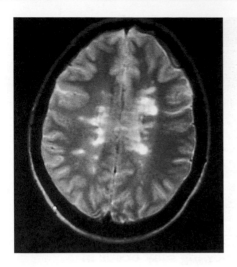

28   Q. MS – true or false?

a. It is an idiopathic, remitting, demyelinating disease involving grey matter within the CNS.

b. Presentation with progressive disease is the most common.

c. Lumbar puncture shows leucocytosis, IgG level >15% of total protein and oligoclonal bands on protein electrophoresis.

d. Acute demyelination plaques may be highlighted with gadolinium on T2-weighted imaging.

e. Uhthoff phenomenon describes sudden worsening of vision or other symptoms on exercise or increase in body temperature.

f. The long-term prognosis is universally poor.

A.

a. False – white matter. **b.** False – relapsing remitting disease is far more common. **c.** True. **d.** False – T1-weighted (see above). **e.** True. **f.** False.

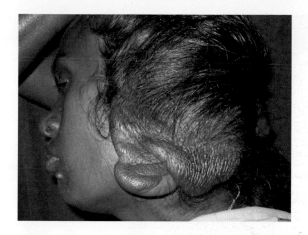

29 Q. Neurofibromatosis-1 – true or false?

a. Inheritance is AD with the gene locus on 17q11.

b. 'Café-au-lait' spots appear during the end of the first decade.

c. Intracranial tumours are primarily meningiomas and gliomas.

d. Elephantiasis nervosa (see above) is associated with nodular plexiform neurofibromas.

e. Most patients eventually develop Lisch nodules.

f. Phaeochromocytoma develops in 15% of patients.

A.

a. True. **b.** False – appear during the first year of life. **c.** True. **d.** False – with diffuse plexiform neurofibromas. **e.** True. **f.** False.

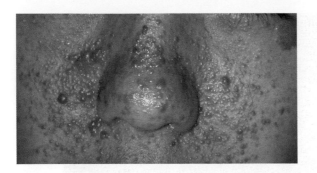

30 Q. Other phacomatoses – true or false?

a. Adenoma sebaceum (see above) is present in 70% of patients with tuberous sclerosis.

b. Shagreen patches in tuberous sclerosis consist of diffuse thickening over the sternum.

c. Inheritance of Sturge–Weber syndrome is AD.

d. Bisystem Sturge–Weber syndrome involves the face and eyes or the face and leptomeninges.

e. CNS haemangioblastoma in von Hippel–Lindau syndrome occurs in about 25% of patients with retinal tumours.

f. Polycythaemia in von Hippel–Lindau syndrome may be the result of factors released by a cerebellar or renal tumour.

A.

a. False – it is universal. **b.** False – over the lumbar region. **c.** False – it is sporadic. **d.** True. **e.** True. **f.** True.

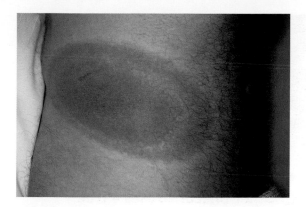

31 **Q. Match the skin lesion (a–f) with the appropriate disease (i–vi).**

a. Erythema nodosum.

b. Erythema chronicum migrans (see above).

c. Leopard skin.

d. Condylomata lata.

e. Vitiligo.

f. Dermatographia.

i. Behçet syndrome.

ii. Vogt–Koyanagi–Harada syndrome.

iii. Onchocerciasis.

iv. Lyme disease.

v. Sarcoidosis.

vi. Syphilis.

A.

a. & **v**; **b.** & **iv**; **c.** & **iii**; **d.** & **vi**; **e.** & **ii**; **f.** & **i**.

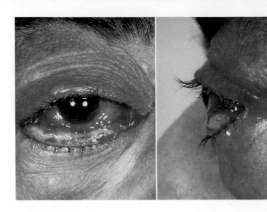

32   Q. Match the autoimmune disorder (a–f) with the appropriate ophthalmic manifestation (i–vi).

a. Sjögren syndrome.

b. Sympathetic ophthalmia.

c. Vogt–Koyanagi–Harada syndrome.

d. Cicatrical pemphigoid.

e. Cogan syndrome.

f. Wegener granulomatosis.

i. Exudative retinal detachment.

ii. Dalen–Fuchs nodules.

iii. Interstitial keratitis.

iv. Punctate epitheliopathy.

v. Symblepharon.

vi. Orbital inflammatory disease (see above).

A.

a. & **iv**; **b.** & **ii**; **c.** & **i**; **d.** & **v**; **e.** & **iii**; **f.** and **vi**.

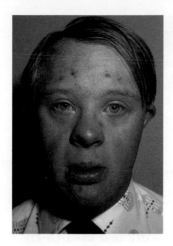

33 **Q. Match the corneal changes (a–f) with appropriate systemic condition (i–vi).**

a. Crystalline keratopathy.

b. Vortex keratopathy.

c. Kayser–Fleischer ring.

d. Corneal pseudodendrites.

e. Band keratopathy.

f. Keratoconus.

i. Fabry disease.

ii. Wilson disease.

iii. Cystinosis.

iv. Hypercalcaemia.

v. Tyrosinaemia.

vi. Down syndrome (see above).

A.

a. & **iii**; **b.** & **i**; **c.** & **ii**; **d.** & **v**; **e.** & **iv**; **f.** & **vi**.

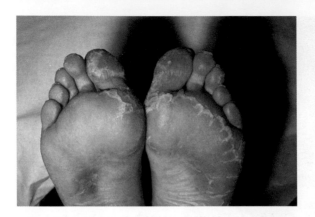

34 **Q. Match the following diseases (a–d) with the appropriate HLA (i–iv).**

a. Behçet syndrome.

b. Reiter syndrome (see above).

c. Vogt–Koyanagi–Harada syndrome.

d. Type 1 diabetes.

i. HLA-B51

ii. HLA-DR1 and DR4.

iii. HLA-B27.

iv. HLA-DR3.

A.

a. & **i**; **b.** & **iii**; **c.** & **ii**; **d.** & **iv**.

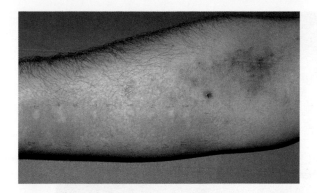

35 Q. The following may be associated with cataract – true or false?

a. Diabetes mellitus.

b. Neurofibromatosis-1.

c. Myotonic dystrophy.

d. Polycythaemia rubra vera.

e. Atopic dermatitis (see above).

f. Cushing syndrome.

A.

a. True. **b.** False – neurofibromatosis-2. **c.** True. **d.** False. **e.** True.
f. True.

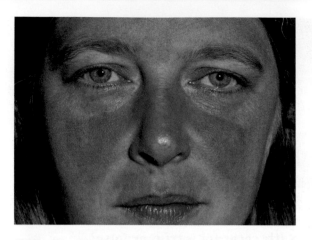

36   **Q. Match the autoimmune disorder (a–d) with the appropriate serum autoantibodies (i–iv).**

a. Wegener granulomatosis.

b. Systemic lupus erythematosus (see above).

c. Myasthenia gravis.

d. Systemic sclerosis.

i. Antinuclear antibodies against double-stranded DNA (ds DNA).

ii. Antinuclear antibodies against single-stranded DNA (ss DNA).

iii. Autoantibodies against granulocyte cytoplasm (c ANCA).

iv. Antibodies against acetylcholine receptors.

A.

a. & **iii**; **b.** & **i**; **c.** & **iv**; **d.** & **ii**.

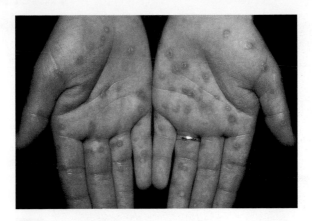

37

Q. Match the investigation (a–f) with the appropriate disease (i–vi).

a. Angiotensin converting enzyme.

b. Sabin–Feldman.

c. MHA-TP.

d. HLA tissue typing.

i. Toxoplasmosis.

ii. Syphilis (see above).

iii. Reiter syndrome.

iv. Sarcoidosis.

A.

a. & **ii**; **b.** & **i**: **c.** & **vi**; **d.** & **iii**.

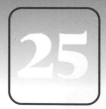
Immediate referral

The following conditions should be referred very urgently (no more than a few hours) because they pose a risk of permanent blindness or serious health problems. Rare conditions that the optometrist is most unlikely to encounter have not been included.

Anterior segment

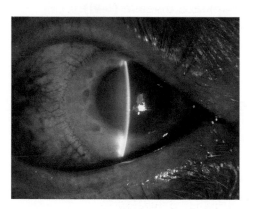

1. Acute angle-closure glaucoma

- More common in women.
- Past history of haloes are suggestive of subacute angle closure attacks.
- Pain, corneal haze, shallow anterior chamber and a dilated and unreactive pupil to light (see above).
- Good prognosis with prompt treatment.

NB: Prophylactic laser iridotomy is required to the fellow eye.

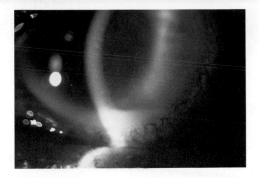

2. Acute postoperative endophthalmitis

- Typically occurs within 4 days of intraocular surgery – usually cataract.
- Patient would have been discharged from hospital.
- Painful eye with a white fluid level in the anterior chamber (hypopyon – see above).
- Guarded prognosis even with prompt treatment.

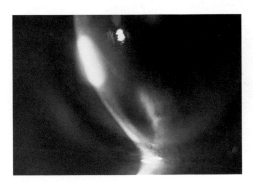

3. Bacterial keratitis

- Painful red eye with a white corneal infiltrate (see above).
- Hypopyon in very severe cases.
- May be associated with contact lens wear.
- Good prognosis if treated early.

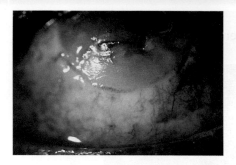

4. Severe chemical burn

- Severe pain.
- Corneal oedema and conjunctival ischaemia (see above).
- Guarded prognosis.

NB: Optometrist must immediately irrigate the eye with water for 15 minutes before referring the patient.

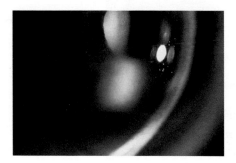

5. Large hyphaema

- History of blunt trauma.
- Red fluid level in the anterior chamber (see above).
- Relatively good prognosis.

NB: Secondary haemorrhage may occur after a few days.

Posterior segment

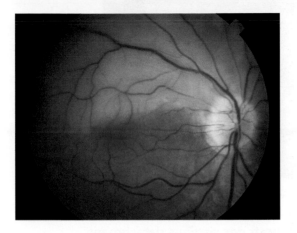

1. Retinal artery occlusion

- Sudden, painless, unilateral visual loss.
- Visual acuity depends on the severity of occlusion (i.e. involving a branch or the central retinal artery).
- Pale fundus with stagnation of arterial blood column (see above).
- Visual prognosis in most cases is very poor but occasionally prompt treatment may be successful.

2. Arteritic anterior ischaemic optic neuropathy

- Sudden, unilateral visual loss in an elderly patient.
- Important associated symptoms of giant-cell arteritis are headache and pain in the jaws while chewing.
- Pale, swollen disc with peripapillary haemorrhages (see below).
- Very poor visual prognosis despite prompt treatment.

NB: Blindness in the other eye can frequently be prevented by systemic steroids.

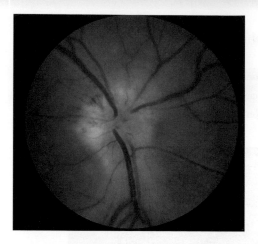

3. Acute posterior vitreous detachment

- Sudden onset of unilateral flashes and floaters.
- Vitreous blood may be present.
- About 10% of patients have a retinal tear which must be treated prophylactically with laser (see below) to prevent retinal detachment.

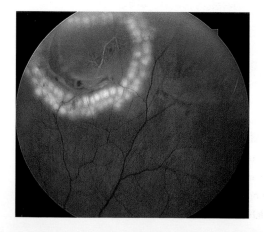

Neurological emergencies

The following conditions are associated with a high risk of stroke and should be referred to the general practitioner or a neurologist, and not to an ophthalmologist.

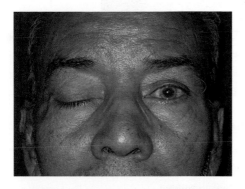

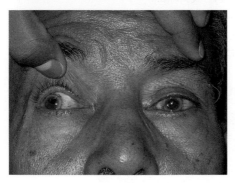

1. Acute third nerve palsy
- Important to exclude life-threatening intracranial aneurysm which may rupture at any time and result in death.
- Ptosis and ophthalmoplegia (see above).

NB: Pain and a fixed dilated pupil are suggestive of aneurysm.

2. Transient retinal ischaemic attacks

- Recurrent attacks of painless unilateral visual loss, often described as a curtain coming over the eye, usually from top to bottom, lasting a few minutes.
- Frequency of attacks varies from several times a day to once every few months.
- Caused by retinal embolization, usually from carotid artery disease.
- Antiplatelet therapy is required to reduce the risk of permanent retinal artery occlusion or stroke.

NB: Fundus examination is usually normal between attacks.

Urgent referral

1. Severe disc new vessels in proliferative diabetic retinopathy.
2. Suspected choroidal melanoma.
3. Recent vitreous haemorrhage.
4. Recent onset of diplopia in an adult.
5. Recent onset of metamorphopsia.

Non-urgent referral

1. Macular hole.
2. Retinal vein occlusion.
3. Suspected open-angle glaucoma.
4. Squint in a child.
5. Severe background diabetic retinopathy.
6. Pre-proliferative diabetic retinopathy.

Do not refer

1. Subconjunctival haemorrhage.
2. Congenital hypertrophy of the retinal pigment epithelium.
3. Peripheral pavingstone degeneration.
4. Mild background diabetic retinopathy.
5. Early cataract without visual problems.
6. Patients with migraine.
7. Macular drusen and normal visual acuity.

Index